MIDLIFE CAN WAIT

MIDLIFE CAN WAIT

HOW TO STAY YOUNG and HEALTHY AFTER 35

BERNARD A. ESKIN, M.D.
and LYNNE S. DUMAS

BALLANTINE BOOKS • NEW YORK

Sale of this book without a front cover may be unauthorized. If this book is coverless, it may have been reported to the publisher as "unsold or destroyed" and neither the author nor the publisher may have received payment for it.

Copyright © 1995 by Bernard A. Eskin, M.D. and Lynne S. Dumas

All rights reserved under International and Pan-American Copyright Conventions. Published in the United States by Ballantine Books, a division of Random House, Inc., New York, and simultaneously in Canada by Random House of Canada Limited, Toronto.

Library of Congress Catalog Card Number: 94-94561

ISBN: 0-345-37652-8

Cover design by Ruth Ross
Text design by Debby Jay

Manufactured in the United States of America

First Edition: March 1995

10 9 8 7 6 5 4 3 2 1

This work is dedicated to my wife, Lynn, whose transitional years inspired me.

Dr. Bernard A. Eskin

Contents

Acknowledgments ix
Authors' Note xi

Introduction 3
1. Who Is the Transitional Woman? 9
2. Natural Ways to Maximize Your Vitality 25
3. Coping with Menstrual Changes 48
4. Hot Flashes . . . At *Your* Age? 76
5. Birth Control After Thirty-Five 100
6. How to Enhance—and Stretch—Your Fertility 120
7. How to Enjoy the Best Sex Ever 158
8. Managing Estrogen- and Age-Related Medical Conditions 191
9. The Thyroid: Outsmarting a Midlife Imposter 215
10. Beating Serious Illness 234
11. A Doctor's Guide to Looking Good 263
12. Finding Emotional Well-being 282

Appendix A: Biology 101: The Female Reproductive Cycle 306
Appendix B: A Guide to Medical Tests 314
Bibliography 318
Index 327

Acknowledgments

Our thanks go to many people, but especially Herb and Nancy Katz for their faith and energy in keeping this project going despite the hurdles that appeared; Joëlle Delbourgo for her enthusiasm, guidance, and patience; and Nellie Sabin for her editorial savvy.

We'd also like to thank these organizations for their input: the American Cancer Society, the American College of Obstetricians and Gynecologists, the American Fertility Society, the American Heart Association, the National Alliance of Breast Cancer Organizations, the National Cancer Institute, and the National Thyroid Foundation.

And, from Lynne: "A special thanks to my husband, Dominick Scotto, for offering safe harbor and never-ending support."

Authors' Note

Throughout this book you will find many stories of midlife women. These are composite sketches of several women created in order to protect the privacy of my patients. The medical information, however, remains accurate.

Midlife Can Wait

Introduction

From the Doctor ...

Women between the ages of thirty-six and fifty—what I call *the transitional years*—often come to see me feeling confused and upset by the changes their bodies are undergoing. They don't understand what they are experiencing—whether these changes are harmless annoyances or serious health problems—and they're angry that they feel so helpless and out of control.

The transitional years form a unique stage for women, but for years doctors didn't pay much attention to the special needs of women of this age. Since many physicians believed that women in their late thirties or their forties were no longer all that concerned about childbearing and not yet bothered by menopause, they considered this stage of life "easy." But what this means is that for too long the medical needs of an important and, thanks to the baby boom, enormous group of women have been both misunderstood and ignored.

I want to change all that. I want women to know that the transitional years constitute a very distinct stage of life. Specifically, I want to make sure they understand four key points.

- First, that the changes taking place in their bodies are a natural and normal result of heading toward menopause, the next major point along life's continuum.
- Second, that enormous variation exists in how these changes take place in individual women.
- Third, that while most changes are harmless, some do signal trouble and require medical attention.
- And fourth, perhaps most importantly, that there is much transitional women can do, not only to cope with these changes but also to delay or even prevent them, thus ensuring that they maintain their health and vitality—and continue to feel terrific—for years to come.

What's more, after spending thirty years as a practicing gynecologist and reproductive endocrinologist researching and working with women between the ages of thirty-six and fifty, I am absolutely convinced that transitional women can keep menopause at bay for a good, long time. It's all a matter of understanding how your body is changing and aging, so that you can do whatever is necessary—from modifying your diet to avoiding unnecessary gynecological surgery—to maintain and even improve your health, vigor, and energy now and in the years ahead.

You can also counteract many of the common complaints associated with the transitional years. For instance, many women concerned about the winding down of their biological clock are completely successful in extending their fertility! In addition, if you heed the recommendations I offer in the chapters that follow, you'll be able to cut dramatically your risk for osteoporosis, thyroid disorder, heart disease, and a host of other potentially serious health problems that can threaten your vitality and youthful well-being.

By the time you finish reading this book, you may actually know more about women's health than some doctors. I hope, then, that you will arm yourself with the information

Introduction

offered and insist that your doctor take your age-related changes and concerns seriously. After all, your best years still lie ahead!

And from the Transitional Woman ...

On the morning of my thirtieth birthday, I dragged myself into the bathroom, peered into the mirror—and discovered my first gray hair. I was not pleased. I suppose it was one of Mother Nature's cruel little jokes.

Okay. I could deal with this. What's a gray hair or two? Nothing my hairdresser couldn't fix. Besides, it didn't *mean* anything, did it? My mother had turned gray when she was very young, so it was not surprising that I would, too.

Despite this inauspicious event, the rest of my thirtieth year and the five after that turned out to be pretty terrific. My whole life began falling into place. I married a wonderful man, found a great apartment, and achieved some measure of the professional success I'd always wanted. I discovered that "color highlighting" would take care of that pesky gray hair. And to insure that my body would otherwise behave itself, I embarked on a sound health regimen.

I began exercising regularly and eliminated red meat, caffeine, and a good deal of fat from my diet. I started eating more healthful foods, like legumes and whole grain breads. (My husband always teases me, however, that my quest for good health stops mysteriously short of giving up chocolate.) Since I'd never smoked and rarely drank, no changes were necessary there, but I started keeping my weight under better control. As long as I had anything to say about it—and I was convinced that I'd have a good deal to say about it for many, many years—I was determined to stay as youthful and healthy as I'd always been.

Which is why I was so unnerved—and annoyed—when at age thirty-six, just when I seemed to have gotten my life all together, my body started falling apart.

First, my periods became less regular. I had always been able to set my watch by my twenty-eight-day cycles. Now I found myself increasingly surprised, often inconvenienced, and sometimes even embarrassed by an early- or late-appearing period that was shorter but more intense than before. I also began suffering from what I self-diagnosed as premenstrual syndrome (PMS). A week or so before my period, my breasts would get incredibly tender, I'd bloat up like a water balloon, and my anxiety level would soar. Deadlines I once deemed manageable seemed impossible to meet; planning a simple dinner for a few friends became an overwhelming task that I felt I could never pull off—until I started to menstruate, at which time everything seemed workable again.

I also noticed that I had less energy. I used to be able to party well into a Saturday night; now, I found myself looking forward to staying home, renting a video, and calling out for a pizza. Always a morning person, I used to get up early, grab a muffin, and plunge right into my work. Now, I found I'd have to ease myself into the day, sipping my herbal tea and thumbing through the newspaper for an hour or so before I could get started. Since I also fell asleep earlier, I found my productive time shortened, which made it more difficult to accomplish all my very full life demanded.

Then I discovered something else: I wasn't alone. My closest friends, all of whom were around my age, confided that they, too, were experiencing some puzzling and sometimes disturbing changes. They felt as bewildered and frustrated as I did, frequently asking themselves, "What the

Introduction

heck is going on here? We're doing everything the experts recommend—exercising, eating right—and we're still losing ground. All our lives we've believed that we could always be in charge of our bodies, our selves. We belong to the generation that would outsmart growing old. So what is happening to us?"

Somehow our bodies just weren't behaving the way we expected. Our periods were changing, our skin was becoming drier, our sex drive was wilting, our energy diminishing. Surely we were too young for middle age and menopause. Our friends were still having their first babies, for God's sake!

The other possibility, the one we whispered to each other in our most vulnerable moments, was that the changes we were experiencing weren't normal. Couldn't a sudden midcycle bleed be a sign of cancer? Mightn't a lack of energy be due to some awful blood disorder? Could a decreased libido be caused by some terribly malfunctioning gland?

The answers eluded us. So my friends and I began reading everything we could find on women's health. But we could find scarcely any information on the changes that women in our age group—that is, mid-to-late thirties and forties—were experiencing.

Then I learned of the work being done by Dr. Bernard A. Eskin. A professor of obstetrics and gynecology at The Medical College of Pennsylvania, he not only has a thriving practice as a gynecologist and fertility specialist in Philadelphia but also has spent many years studying menopause. In fact, he'd written one of the most respected textbooks on the subject and was considered one of the nation's leading experts. But what most interested me was that he'd also conducted extensive research studies on women who had not yet reached menopause, women between the ages of thirty-six and fifty.

I managed to get a few of Dr. Eskin's professional articles and a couple of little blurbs in popular magazines that mentioned his work. And that's when I began to get excited. It appeared that Dr. Eskin knew all about the changes and problems women my age were encountering. So I decided that I had to find him.

Well, when at last we met, I was blown away. First of all, this brilliant doctor, whose list of professional credentials boasts twelve books and innumerable professional honors, is a sweet, unpretentious, avuncular gentleman who immediately insisted I call him Bernie. (I soon learned that everyone, even his patients, calls him that.) As Bernie began to talk about his work, I realized how much he liked women and how sensitive he was to their problems and concerns, particularly women in my age group.

Bernie had a lot to say about the transitional years. He'd begun doing research on women ages thirty-six to fifty back in the seventies, and had published numerous papers in medical journals on transitional women's sexuality, fertility (and infertility), menstrual changes, and thyroid problems. I also learned that he had been toying with the idea of writing a book for transitional women that would get his ideas and research findings out to an audience larger than the professional medical community and the transitional women he'd treated in his private practice. That's when my journalistic instincts kicked in.

Bernie and I soon began collaborating; what you are about to read is the special result of our work. So if you're a woman between thirty-six and fifty who hasn't yet reached menopause, read on. This book is just for you!

1

Who Is the Transitional Woman?

- The Transitional Woman
- Aging and Estrogen: An Overview
- Age-Related Changes You May Experience
- Psychological and Psychosocial Change

Tears came into Susan's eyes as she explained, "I can't believe this is happening to me. I'm thirty-nine, finally ready to have a baby—you know Mark and I put it off for a few years—but we're not getting anywhere. We've been trying to get pregnant for eight months and we haven't had any luck.

"Maybe it's because my periods have become incredibly irregular. I can't figure out the best time to conceive because my cycle keeps changing. I'm also noticing other changes which are getting me down, like my hair's getting grayer and I can't seem to control my weight. I feel anxious all the time, and depressed—plus, I'll be forty in two months.

Forty! How did this happen to me? I know everyone grows older . . . but I'm not ready for middle age!"

I've asked hundreds of women between thirty-six and forty-nine how old they feel, and almost without exception they name a number that's about ten years younger than their chronological age. In part, this is because as a culture we have a distorted idea of what "midlife" means. Many women think growing older means sagging breasts, thicker waistlines, dowdy clothes, lukewarm sex, and, of course, menopause. If that's your view, then of course you're not ready for midlife!

Even though menopause is getting better press these days—happily, some of our most respected feminist authors are urging women to reassess menopause, to view it not as an end but as the beginning of the second, and often best, half of your life—the unenlightened fact of the matter is that no one feels she's "ready" to make the transition into menopause. Instead, she wants to stay as vigorous and youthful as she's always been for as long as is humanly possible.

Well, get ready to smile, because I'm here to tell you that these transitional years can be filled with good health and high spirits. Certain changes are inevitable, but there are steps you can take to keep up your energy level, minimize age-related complaints, and avoid serious illness. This all adds up to many more youthful, productive years.

The Transitional Woman

In the many years that I've practiced medicine, I've heard all the myths surrounding menopause. One persistent and totally misleading idea is that menopause hits with an unexpected thud—that it's a catastrophic event you suddenly confront when you wake up one morning. Nothing could be further from the truth.

Menopause is simply the *final* cessation of your periods. It does not occur suddenly or without warning. In fact—and I have spent thousands of hours treating and studying women to understand this fully—your body starts preparing itself for menopause years earlier than was previously thought. You actually begin making the *transition* from the childbearing to the menopausal years at about age thirty-six. This means you may go through some fifteen years of physiological changes or "preparation" before you finally stop having your periods and enter menopause. Since most women reach menopause at about age fifty-one, I believe we need to think of the ten to fifteen years of typically gradual but occasionally dramatic changes as "transitional years," and women between the ages of thirty-six and fifty as "transitional women."

Thanks to the postwar baby boom, an unprecedented number of women, born between 1946 and 1964, are now smack in the middle of their transitional years. In 1993 over 29 million American women were between the ages of thirty-six to fifty.

Transitional women share many characteristics. Among the most notable are the physical, age-related changes they experience, the *biological markers* common to women in their transitional years. The most significant are:

- *A decrease in the effectiveness of the ovaries.* During transition the ovaries begin to secrete less estrogen, which, as I will explain shortly, has an enormous impact on how your body functions—including increasing the possibility of hot flashes. Additionally, the transitional woman's ovaries contain fewer and older eggs, which makes fertility problems more likely.

- *Changes in your menstrual cycle.* Your periods may become shorter or longer, less or more intense, thanks to the shifting hormonal balances of your system.
- *A decrease in bone strength.* Transitional women may begin to experience a slight reduction in bone mass, which can make bones weaker and more brittle.
- *A decline in muscle tone and strength,* particularly for women who do not exercise regularly and eat a well-balanced diet.
- *Fewer secretions of the hair and skin follicles,* which can lead to hair and skin dryness.
- *Fewer secretions of the mucous membranes of the vagina,* which can cause vaginal dryness and lead to discomfort during sexual intercourse.

All transitional women experience these changes to some degree, although there is *enormous* variation from individual to individual. For some lucky women, the changes are nearly imperceptible. For example, their menstrual cycles may actually be shorter, but only by a day or so, and not every month at that, so that they don't even notice. Other women have such dense bones to begin with that the start of any reduction in mass has little discernible impact on their bone strength. These fortunate individuals glide through their transitional years almost completely unaffected and move into menopause with little or no discomfort.

But for most transitional women, the changes their bodies undergo bring at least some measure of distress. At age thirty-eight, for example, Carla's periods "suddenly" became so unpredictable and heavy that twice they started in the middle of an important company meeting at the ad agency where she is an account executive, causing her much embarrassment as well as physical discomfort.

"I couldn't believe it. There I sat, in the middle of a presentation to one of our most important clients, and all of a sudden I felt something uncomfortable. I look down and my pale blue silk skirt has this huge, red stain. My period wasn't due for four days! Let me tell you, I wanted to crawl under the conference table and die."

It's estimated that 60 percent of transitional women suffer problems irritating or alarming enough to propel them into their doctors' offices for treatment or advice. My belief is that this percentage is probably low, because transitional women's problems are often underreported or even unrecognized by doctors.

If a thirty-six-year-old woman complains of hot flashes, for example, her doctor may simply dismiss them as a product of her imagination because the doctor was taught (and wrongly so) that hot flashes are only an issue for older, menopausal women. Yes, doctors are becoming better informed as we learn more about the special needs of women in their transitional years. But this troublesome situation is not changing fast enough, particularly for those of you suffering from upsetting symptoms right now.

AGING AND ESTROGEN: AN OVERVIEW

The natural aging process lies behind the changes you're experiencing. As you grow older, overall cell activity decreases, causing you to tire more easily and to take longer to feel refreshed. Muscle tone may not be as good as it once was, particularly if you don't exercise regularly. Cuts and bruises may take longer to heal, and bowels may slow, resulting in more frequent bouts of constipation. At about age forty, vision usually begins to change; often, you become presbyopic. (I call presbyopia "long-arm syndrome," because you go to a restaurant, pick up the menu, and have to stretch your arms out as far in front of you as possible so you can read it.)

In addition to a kind of generalized cell slowdown experienced by both men and women, women must contend with another problem: at about age thirty-five or thirty-six, their ovaries begin to decrease their production of the powerful female sex hormone, estrogen.

At the risk of oversimplification, think of estrogen as the hormone that differentiates women from men. Estrogen keeps a woman's reproductive organs in good working order and affects the health of the vagina, vulva, uterus, bladder, urethra, skin, hair, mucous membranes, bones, heart and blood vessels, pelvic muscles, and brain. This single potent hormone promotes full breasts, smooth skin, thick shiny hair, and strong bones. It also plays a role in keeping your cholesterol count in check.

Up until quite recently, doctors thought that estrogen levels peaked at about age twenty-seven and declined slightly after that, leveling off at about age thirty-five and staying relatively stable until age forty-six to fifty, the years just prior to menopause, when there would be a radical drop. But a study I conducted, the results of which I presented in the spring of 1993 at a national meeting of the American College of Obstetricians and Gynecologists, revealed a very different—and quite astonishing—finding. As figure 1 shows, while estrogen does peak at about age twenty-seven, it levels off only until about age thirty-five. But between ages thirty-five and forty-six, estrogen levels drop steadily and fairly dramatically. In fact, by the time you reach age forty-two, the mean amount of estrogen produced by your body is one-third less than what it was fifteen years earlier. Estrogen levels continue to drop, reaching a significantly lower point at

Who Is the Transitional Woman?

about age fifty-one, the average age of menopause, and hitting their nadir by your late sixties.

FIGURE 1. *Lifetime Estrogen Levels*

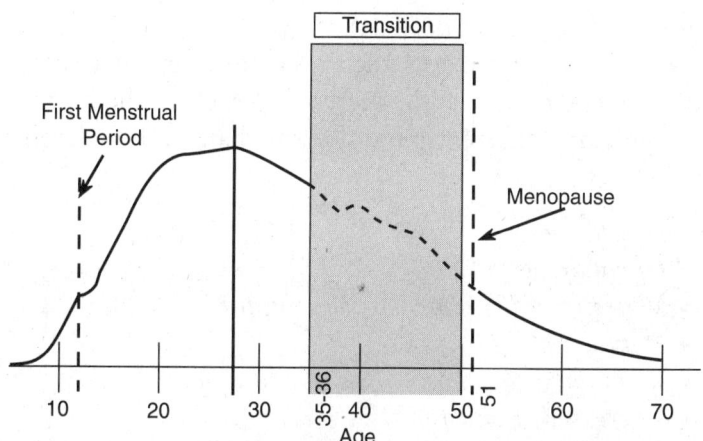

It is important to emphasize that I am talking about mean, or average, estrogen levels here. You see, as you move through your transitional years, the amount of estrogen necessary to bring about ovulation during any given cycle increases more dramatically than it did when you were younger. But as soon as ovulation occurs (and the second half of your cycle begins), estrogen drops to a much lower level than it did when you were younger. As a result, the *mean* amount of estrogen that you have during a given cycle is lower than it was prior to the transitional years. Figure 1 illustrates these mean estrogen levels.

(FYI: You will notice that there's a slight blip on this figure showing a temporary hike in estrogen at around age forty. Here's why. After age thirty-seven, your ovaries lose some of their ability to produce adequate estrogen. Your pituitary and hypothalamus glands recognize this situation and try to come to the rescue by triggering the release of more FSH [follicle-stimulating hormone], which will stimulate the ovaries to produce more estrogen. This works for a while, but eventually your ovaries tire and estrogen levels continue their steady decline.)

Because estrogen exerts such a powerful influence over a woman's body and health, decreasing levels of the hormone result in many different physiological changes. Low levels of estrogen can cause:

- *Hot flashes*
- *Irregular periods*
- *Worsening of premenstrual symptoms*
- *Depression*
- *Irritability*
- *Decreased desire for sex*
- *Vaginal dryness*
- *Memory loss*
- *Skin dryness*

Figure 2 shows the changes in the intensity of these symptoms for a hypothetical "average" woman as estrogen levels start to dip. Keep in mind, however, that every woman is unique; some lose estrogen faster or more slowly than average. Nonetheless, this graph can help you get some idea of what typically occurs as a woman's estrogen level drops.

Who Is the Transitional Woman?

FIGURE 2. *Intensity of Certain Transitional Symptoms with Age*

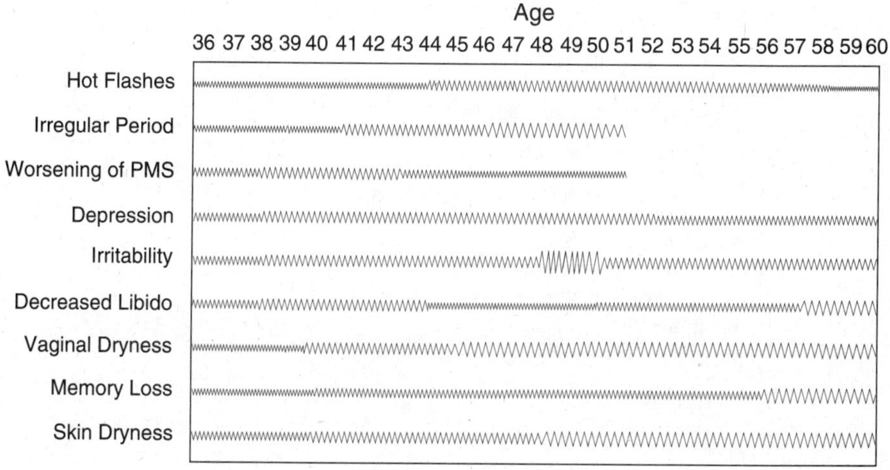

Symptom	36 37 38 39 40 41 42 43 44 45 46 47 48 49 50 51 52 53 54 55 56 57 58 59 60
Hot Flashes	
Irregular Period	
Worsening of PMS	
Depression	
Irritability	
Decreased Libido	
Vaginal Dryness	
Memory Loss	
Skin Dryness	

AGE-RELATED CHANGES YOU MAY EXPERIENCE

As you may suspect, not all age-related changes women encounter occur at once or with the same intensity. Because the transitional phase spans so many years, certain changes are likely to occur early on, while others appear much later, as table 1 shows. Women between thirty-five and thirty-nine, for example, are only slightly likely to suffer a hot flash. But by the time you reach age forty-five, your chances skyrocket.

Sometimes, however, growing older works in your favor. If you suffer from PMS, you're most likely to find your symptoms getting worse when you're between forty and

TABLE 1. *Signs and Symptoms Commonly Encountered in the Transitional Years*

Key:
0   = unlikely
−   = slightly likely
+   = somewhat likely
++ = very likely
+++ = highly likely

Sign/symptom	35–39	40–44	45–50
Vaginal dryness	−	+	++
Vaginal yeast infection	+	+	+
Recurrent urinary tract infection	+	++	++
Reduced sexual vaginal secretions	−	+	++
Irregular periods	+	++	++
Premenstrual symptoms	+	++	+
Hot flashes	−	+	+++
Reduced muscle tone	−	+	++
Skin dryness	+	++	+++
Varicose veins	+	++	++
Cellulite	+	+	+
Slower skin healing	−	+	++
Decreased libido	++	++	+
Thyroid problems	−	++	++
Rise in cholesterol	−	+	++
Breast hair	−	+	+
Sagging breasts	−	+	++
Fibrocystic disease	+	++	+
Facial hair	−	+	+
Graying hair	+	++	+++
Thinning hair	0	−	+
Dandruff	+	++	+++
Reduced stamina	+	++	+++
Constipation	−	+	++
Eye dryness	0	−	+
Vision problems	−	+	++
Bone loss	−	+	++
Increased sweating	−	+	++
Short-term memory loss	−	+	++
Breaks in concentration	+	++	++
Headaches	−	+	+
Irritability	+	++	+++
Depression	+	+++	++
Mood swings	+	+++	++
Anxiety	+	+++	++

forty-four. By the time you're forty-five, however, you can expect your PMS problems to ease. Eventually, they'll disappear completely.

There's too much individual variation to predict precisely what you will encounter in your transitional years. However, here are a few of the most widespread and significant problems.

- *Changes in your menstrual cycle.* Changes in your monthly cycle are one of the earliest and most common symptoms of the transitional years. They may be quite subtle when you're in your thirties, but usually become more obvious as you grow older. Your periods may become much lighter, heavier, shorter, or longer. In most cases, such changes are perfectly normal and no cause for alarm. But some changes, such as severe menstrual cramping and/or excessive, dark blood flow may require medical attention. (For more information on the menstrual changes transitional women may experience, see Chapter Three.)
- *Hot flashes.* The latest research shows that it's not unusual for women as young as thirty-six or thirty-seven to feel a sudden burst of intense heat (usually followed by a cold sweat) known as a hot flash. The good news: if hot flashes bother you, they can be treated easily through diet, exercise, and medication. (See Chapter Four for a more detailed exploration of hot flashes in the transitional years.)
- *Reduced stamina.* Many transitional women find they tire more easily than they did when they were younger. There's a reason for that. When you're physically active, your muscles produce lactic acid and other chemicals; to get rid of the acid and revitalize the muscles, your body needs a short period of rest. As you get older, it takes your body longer to remove the chemicals from your muscles, so you need to rest sooner, more frequently, and for a bit

longer than you did when you were younger. True, regular, rigorous exercise can build up your stamina. But even a forty-year-old athlete would be hard-pressed to outlast her twenty-year-old rival, no matter what shape she's in.

• *Bone loss.* Bone mass—and thus, bone strength—often decline after age forty-five. There are at least three reasons why:

1. The natural aging process may prevent the intestines from absorbing enough calcium; thus, the calcium you need to maintain bone mass may not be available in your blood.

2. In order for your body to metabolize calcium and form new bone, you need a good supply of active vitamin D (D_3). But since you need estrogen to form this vitamin, and since transitional women have less estrogen in their system, their ability to form new bone is reduced. (For more on how vitamin D_3 works, see Chapter Eight.)

3. When estrogen and progesterone levels are low, more calcium may be lost during urination, thus hastening the development of brittle bones.

There may be other reasons for bone loss as well. Recent research, most notably a 1990 study conducted at the University of Denmark, suggests that receptors for estrogen may actually exist in bone. When estrogen levels decline, then, so would receptor activity, causing reduced bone mass, or weaker bones.

• *Short-term memory loss.* If you find yourself having more trouble remembering where you put the car keys or recalling the name of the actor who starred in the movie you watched last night, you probably don't have an early case of Alzheimer's. Instead, you can chalk up these lapses to "neurogenic aging symptoms" (NAS), a term I coined to refer to age-related changes in the way your nerves work. Among other symptoms, NAS can bring about memory loss, particularly after age forty. (For more information on NAS, see Chapter Eight.)

- *PMS.* Even if you've never been bothered by premenstrual syndrome before, you may now find yourself feeling anxious, depressed, bloated, or suffering with sore, tender breasts a week or so before your period. Doctors believe that a sudden shift in the delicate balance between estrogen and progesterone could explain why many women experience more, and more intense, premenstrual symptoms with age.
- *Thyroid problems.* If you've been feeling weak, lethargic, depressed, moody, and generally out of sorts, you may be suffering from a faulty thyroid. Estrogen helps keep the thyroid gland in good working order, so lower estrogen levels may cause the thyroid to become sluggish, resulting in a condition called hypothyroidism, or underactive thyroid, and the symptoms mentioned above.
- *Atrophism.* Atrophism is the medical term for the drying out of areas of both skin and mucous membranes throughout the body, including the scalp, face, and vagina. This is a common and annoying problem of the transitional years.
- *Decreased libido.* Transitional women often complain that they've lost their old sex drive. Lower estrogen levels can cause vaginal dryness, which, in turn, can make intercourse uncomfortable, if not downright painful, turning sex into something to be avoided rather than anticipated. Also, since sex is both a physical and emotional activity, the hectic, pressure-filled life-style of most transitional women leaves them little time, energy, or enthusiasm for sex.
- *Difficulty getting pregnant.* Not every transitional woman wants to have a baby, but among those who do, fertility problems are not unusual.

Psychological and Psychosocial Changes

For better *and* worse, women often go through some amount of emotional upheaval during their transitional years. On the upside, they've survived their turbulent twenties and early thirties and have come out more confident and secure in themselves, in who they are and what they want. By this time, most women also have professional success and/or families, friends, and home lives that bring a deep sense of personal satisfaction.

At the same time, however, many transitional women may feel insecure and upset about growing older in a society obsessed with youth. These negative feelings are, of course, tied to the physical changes they're experiencing. It's common for transitional women to worry or feel down about the unfamiliar and disturbing direction their bodies seem to be taking.

Any sudden physical change—mid-cycle spotting, missing a period, getting hit with an unexpected hot flash—understandably triggers concern. When Sherry, forty-two, missed her period for two months straight and knew she wasn't pregnant, she became alarmed. She worried, "Is what is happening to me serious? Could it be menopause? Cancer? Can it be treated? Cured?" (As we'll see later, skipped periods are common in the transitional years.)

Cosmetic changes, like the appearance of facial hair or those first few "laugh lines," can also make some women feel old, unattractive, and less sexy than they used to feel. Deanna, forty-six, felt her self-esteem crumbling when she overheard her husband's new business partner say, "Is that his wife? But she looks so much *older* than he does."

There are lots more ways that physical changes can undercut your emotional well-being and self-esteem as you grow older:

- *Transitional women who want to have children often have difficulty conceiving,* which can make them feel anxious, depressed, unfeminine, and angry that their bodies have let them down.
- *Poorer energy levels don't give you the stamina you need* to accomplish all you would like to, either personally or professionally. You may end up feeling inadequate and overwhelmed.
- *Uncomfortable sex can lead to intimacy problems* with your partner, who may or may not understand what you are experiencing.
- *Mood swings, caused by a malfunctioning thyroid, or even a slight shift in your hormone mix,* can make you feel happy and upbeat one moment, down and desperate the next, not to mention irritable, edgy, and anxious.

Physical changes aren't the only factors that trip your emotional switch; psychosocial predicaments can also cause you to short-circuit. Consider these dilemmas so common to the transitional years:

- *Transitional women are part of the "sandwich generation"* caught between the demands of raising young kids and caring for aging or ill parents.
- *Many marriages go awry during the transitional years,* so in addition to physical changes, women may be dealing with the pain and stress of divorce.
- *It's stressful to be looking for a mate (if you're single, of course)* when opportunities to meet available, healthy partners are at a premium.
- *Many transitional women are at an important and

stressful professional juncture, trying to crack the glass ceiling after spending ten to twenty years building a career.

- *An extraordinary number of my patients in their transitional years, particularly working mothers, are coping with constant guilt.* These women feel they're in a no-win situation, plagued by guilt when they're at the office ("I should be spending more time with my family") as well as when they're home ("I have so much to do at work").

Between the physical changes and the psychological challenges you're facing, it's clear that moving through the transitional years isn't easy. But you can do it. The chapters that follow will arm you with some simple, practical tips for dealing with the changes you are experiencing or can expect. In the process, you'll become as healthy, vigorous, and confident as you want to be—probably more than you've ever been before—both today and in the many years to come.

2

Natural Ways to Maximize Your Vitality

- Are You at Risk for Early Menopause?
- Bernie's Ten-Point Plan for Peak Health and Vitality

The question transitional women ask me most often, particularly when they hit their forties, is whether the changes they're experiencing—heavier or lighter periods, the arrival of wrinkles or facial hair, perhaps even a sudden hot flash—mean they're heading into early menopause.

Well, this question isn't easy to answer. Your body *is* changing, preparing itself for menopause. But that doesn't mean you're skidding into menopause before your time, or that you have to lose the youthful vigor and attractiveness you've always enjoyed.

Without realizing it, however, you may be speeding up the onset of menopause or exacerbating certain premenopausal problems. Some factors that affect the symptoms you experience during your transitional years are well within your control.

The following quiz will help you determine if you are at risk for early menopause. It also will help you start thinking about the medical and life-style decisions that promote good health and vigor during midlife.

Are You at Risk for Early Menopause?

1. When did your mother stop menstruating?

    A. Before age 40 (10 points)
    B. Between 40 and 45 (5 points)
    C. Over 45 (0 points)
    D. Don't know (2 points)

    Score: _____

2. Do you smoke cigarettes?

    A. Never smoked or quit more than 1 year ago (0 points)
    B. Quit within past year (2 points)
    C. Smoke less than ½ pack daily (10 points)
    D. Smoke more than ½ pack daily (20 points)

    Score: _____

3. Do you eat more than 3 daily servings of milk, yogurt, cheese, or ice cream?

    A. Yes (5 points)
    B. No (0 points)

    Score: _____

Natural Ways to Maximize Your Vitality

4. Are you more than 10 pounds underweight?

    A. Yes (5 points)
    B. No (0 points)

    Score: _____

5. Are you more than 20 percent over your recommended weight? (If you're not sure, check table 2, on page 38.)

    A. Yes (5 points)
    B. No (0 points)

    Score: _____

6. How many children have you borne?

    A. None (5 points)
    B. One or more before age 28 (0 points)
    C. One or more after age 28 (2 points)

    Score: _____

7. How often do you exercise?

    A. I don't exercise (10 points)
    B. I engage in moderate exercise (at least 20 minutes, but less than an hour) one to two times weekly (5 points)
    C. I engage in moderate exercise three to four times weekly (0 points)
    D. I exercise for several hours nearly every day (5 points)

    Score: _____

8. Have you had surgery to remove all or part of an ovary?

    A. Yes   (10 points)
    B. No   (0 points)

                                                   Score: _____

9. Have you had surgery to have your "tubes tied"?

    A. Yes   (5 points)
    B. No   (0 points)

                                                   Score: _____

10. Have you ever been diagnosed with any of the following chronic diseases:

    A. Tuberculosis   (10 points)
    B. Addison's disease   (10 points)
    C. Rheumatoid arthritis   (5 points)
    D. Galactosemia   (20 points)
    E. Diabetes   (10 points)

                                                   Score: _____

11. Have you ever been treated for cancer with chemotherapy or abdominal radiation therapy?

    A. Yes   (15 points)
    B. No   (0 points)

                                                   Score: _____

12. Do you have sexual intercourse 2 times a week or more on average?

    A. Yes   (0 points)
    B. No   (5 points)

                                               Score: _____

13. Have you ever had a sexually transmitted disease? (This does not include yeast infections but does include gonorrhea, syphilis, genital herpes, chlamydia, and Gardnerella vaginalis.)

    A. Yes   (10 points)
    B. No   (0 points)

                                               Score: _____

14. Do you have a way to manage your stress successfully?

    A. Yes   (0 points)
    B. No   (5 points)

                                               Score: _____

15. Do you eat a low-fat diet regularly (or at least most of the time)?

    A. Yes   (0 points)
    B. No   (10 points)

                                               Score: _____

Interpreting Your Score:
Minimal risk of early menopause   5 to 12 points
Moderate risk   13 to 26 points
High risk   26 or more points

Now you have some idea of where you fit on the "risk" continuum. But even if you find yourself in the most vulnerable group, don't panic. Every transitional woman can slash her risk for early menopause and attain her peak vitality and well-being by following a sound health plan—specifically, my "Ten-Point Plan for Peak Health and Vitality," the *first* program tailored specifically to the needs of transitional women. If you follow the suggestions outlined here, I assure you that you'll be able to postpone premature menopause and eliminate, or at the very least ease, any physical and emotional problems the transitional years can bring.

Bernie's Ten-Point Plan for Peak Health and Vitality

1. *Familiarize yourself with the most common symptoms of the transitional years and understand their causes.*

I find that my best-informed patients:

- *Are less likely to* panic over common age-related changes.
- *Are more likely to* recognize symptoms that need medical attention.
- *Are more likely to* take self-help steps to reduce bothersome complaints during their transitional years.
- *Are more likely to* follow my recommendations and advice because they understand what their bodies need.

One of my patients, thirty-eight-year-old Sandra, makes little effort to keep herself up-to-date on health matters. She doesn't bother to exercise regularly or eat a well-balanced diet. About the only concession she makes to staying healthy is seeing me once a year for a Pap test and breast and pelvic exams. Sandra didn't realize that the pain she was experiencing when having sexual intercourse—something she admitted to me only after suffering with (and worrying about) the problem for nearly two years—could be easily remedied.

By contrast, Lena, forty, makes a point of reading health magazines, staying up-to-date on medical matters, and maintaining a good health regimen. I know that she is doing all she can to help herself, which makes it easier for me to help her. When she started feeling discomfort during intercourse, she was only mildly concerned because she knew that as women get older they often experience a decrease in vaginal lubrication that can make penetration painful. After double-checking with me, she went out and bought an over-the-counter lubricating jelly I recommended—and solved the problem immediately.

2. Keep a symptoms diary to track any premenopausal symptoms you are experiencing.

Premenopausal symptoms can sneak up on you, especially if they're subtle and/or you're too busy to think much about them. If you make a point of writing down any physical changes you are experiencing, you may notice patterns that will make it easier for you to target the steps you can take to maximize your well-being. Also, if you make a point of knowing how your body is behaving now, you'll be more likely to recognize any unusual symptoms if and when they arise in the future.

If you are encountering troublesome changes, keep a careful diary of your symptoms and show it to your physician.

SYMPTOMS DIARY

Year	Month	Day 1 2 3 4 5 6 7 8 9 10 11 12 13 14 15 16 17 18 19 20 21 22 23 24 25 26 27 28 29 30 31
	January	
	February	
	March	
	April	
	May	
	June	
	July	
	August	
	September	
	October	
	November	
	December	

Identify on this chart any of the following symptoms you have experienced:

1 Breast tenderness
2 Hot flashes
3 Insomnia
4 Irritability
5 Mood swings

6 Urinary problems
7 Vaginal bleeding
8 Vaginal problems
9 Other

S Spotting
H Heavy
X Regular

Be specific, though; he or she needs to know not only what your transitional symptoms are but also when they are occurring during your cycle. For instance, unexpected bleeding that occurs immediately before you expected your normal period is less worrisome than unexpected bleeding that occurs mid-cycle. So be sure to chart not only what's happening, but when.

The symptoms diary on page 32 will help you track the transitional changes you are experiencing and make it easier for you to get the right treatment to feel your best. Here's how to use it. Each month, put an X in the corresponding box on the day your menstrual period begins and on every day it lasts. Put an H on any days in which your bleeding is extremely heavy, and an S on any day *other than during your period* when you notice any vaginal bleeding. To chart any other changes or symptoms, put the number of the corresponding symptom (for example: 1 for breast tenderness, 5 for mood swings) in the box. You may well have more than one mark in any given box. At the end of each month, you will have a pretty good record of your individual gynecological picture.

3. Get a thyroid checkup.

Though the thyroid gland is no bigger than a walnut, it can cause enormous problems for transitional women. When working normally, the thyroid churns out a hormone called *thyroxine*, which regulates your body's metabolism (that is, the biochemical activities that allow your body to function effectively). When the thyroid manufactures too little thyroxine, this triggers hypothyroidism, causing you to feel less energetic, more sluggish, and possibly depressed. Hypothyroidism can also cause menstrual irregularities and infertility. What's more, it can weaken your libido and make sexual intercourse uncomfortable because of decreased vaginal secretions.

By age fifty, one in ten women will suffer from hypothyroidism. One of the reasons involves the delicate relationship between estrogen and thyroid hormones. As estrogen levels go down, your thyroid hormone requirements may go up. If your thyroid doesn't pump out enough extra hormone to compensate, you may develop hypothyroidism and the loss of stamina that often goes with it.

Since hypothyroidism is often overlooked or misdiagnosed, you should insist that your doctor perform a simple blood test, called a TSH (thyroid stimulating hormone) test, if you're suffering from any of the symptoms I've just mentioned. Even if you feel fine, it's a good idea to have a baseline TSH test at around age forty and another at forty-five. This will help your doctor detect any significant change in your thyroid activity which could signal a potential problem. (For a more thorough discussion of the thyroid, see Chapter Nine.)

4. *Avoid sexually transmitted diseases (STDs).*

Transitional women need to be especially careful about avoiding STDs, particularly if they want to have a child. Although your genes impose some preset limits on the life of your biological clock, certain sexually transmitted diseases, such as gonorrhea, syphilis, chlamydia, and Gardnerella vaginalis, can rob you of your fertility prematurely by causing chronic pelvic problems. It's essential that sexually active women be able to identify and avoid STDs.

Prompt treatment of an STD reduces the likelihood of lasting problems. However, many infections, such as chlamydia or Gardnerella vaginalis, are often so subtle and insidious that only careful screening can detect them. A blood test is needed to diagnose chlamydia and a DNA culture is used to detect gonorrhea. Without accurate detection and aggressive treatment, an STD may damage your fallopian tubes and, in some cases, your ovaries, causing you to become sterile. (For more information on STDs, see Chapter Seven.)

5. Enjoy more—and better—sex!

Flip around the TV stations any evening or peruse the movie listings in your local paper and you'll get the distinct impression that *everyone* is having sex—and loving every minute of it. Well, that may be far from the truth for transitional women.

Women in their transitional years are often on perpetual overload, struggling to meet the demands of kids, careers, partners, and aging parents all at once. By the end of a long day, they're often too worn out to have the energy or inclination for lovemaking.

Their changing biology may also be putting a damper on their sex life. For instance, as estrogen declines, vaginal secretions may decrease, making intercourse physically less comfortable and appealing.

Yet if you're a transitional woman, too little sex can be hazardous to your health. A recent series of studies shows that *women who have more frequent sexual intercourse have fewer hot flashes than women who do not enjoy regular, weekly sexual intimacy!*

Further research shows that women who have regular sex—at least twice weekly—maintain higher levels of estrogen as they get older than women who have sex infrequently or not at all. That means that enjoying an active sex life can help you get many of the benefits that adequate estrogen levels can bring, *including* regular menstrual periods (which increase your chances of keeping your fertility), healthier skin, hair, gums, and more. What's more, good, frequent sex is self-perpetuating; that is, people with happy, active sexual lives seem to maintain their desire for sex longer, which supports the pop maxim "Use it or lose it."

There are other reasons why sexually active women are healthier and more vital than their less libidinous counterparts. Regular sex helps a woman maintain vaginal turgor, that is, adequate vaginal softness, lubrication, and elasticity. In addition, sexual intercourse helps you maintain adequate secretions of the mucous membrane of the vagina and glands of the vulvar area.

My advice: if you're not having regular sex, see if you can figure out why. Is the problem an overdemanding life-style that leaves you with little energy, a physical problem such as vaginal dryness that makes intercourse painful, or simply lack of opportunity? If you possibly can, do something about it. If you're overextended, hire a baby-sitter or housekeeper, or ask a relative or good friend to give you some occasional relief from kids, home, and the office. If chronic exhaustion isn't the culprit, maybe you and your mate are having problems communicating. In that case, try talking with your partner, explaining what you need and enjoy.

Other ways to fire up your sex life: view erotic videotapes, or experiment with some new positions to heighten sexual excitement. Chapter Seven is all about how to have a healthy sex life, but these ideas should give you some idea of what it takes to enjoy sexual intimacy.

One important qualifier: Please don't think I am urging you to "sleep around." In this age of AIDS and other STDs, hopping into bed with the first available partner you find is *very* risky business. You must be *extremely* careful when choosing a sexual companion, making sure your partner is free of any disease, and, during intercourse, always using a latex condom. But if you have a healthy, willing mate, don't relegate sex to a secondary position in your life. It's important enough to your good health to place it high on your list of things to do—and enjoy!

6. Maintain your optimal weight.

When the Duchess of Windsor said, "You can never be too rich or too thin," she only got it half right. You *can* become too skinny for your body type and frame.

Every woman's body was designed to carry some essential fat stores. If your body fat dips below or rises above a certain healthy threshold, your brain automatically produces additional amounts of certain neurohormones (like endorphins or serotonin) that can cause menstruation to come to a halt. Until the body fat is regained (or lost) and the "fatty threshold" is again reached and maintained, ovulation and estrogen production can stop cold. This can cause not only menstrual irregularities but also infertility, bone loss, and hot flashes.

Every woman is different. Your weight depends not only on how much you eat or exercise but also on your genetic makeup, physiology, and body frame. You do, however, have an optimal weight, and you should be able to comfortably maintain it (plus or minus a few pounds) without overeating or dieting. For women, that means taking in about 1,800 calories per day.

Take a look at table 2 on page 38 for the newest suggested weight levels. I think you'll be surprised to discover just how much you can weigh while keeping fit and healthy throughout the transitional years.

TABLE 2. *Guidelines for Healthy Weight*

The U.S. government offers the following guidelines for weight according to age and height.

Height	Weight without clothes or shoes	
	19–34 years	35 years and over
5'	97–128	108–138
5'1"	101–132	111–143
5'2"	104–137	115–148
5'3"	107–141	119–152
5'4"	111–146	122–157
5'5"	114–150	126–162
5'6"	118–155	130–167
5'7"	121–160	134–172
5'8"	125–164	138–178
5'9"	129–169	142–183
5'10"	132–174	146–188
5'11"	136–179	151–194
6'	140–184	155–199

SOURCE: Agriculture Department, Health and Human Services

Even women who have always kept their weight in check often find they have a tougher time once they reach their transitional years. With age, women gain weight faster and lose it much more slowly than they did when they were younger.

One of the main reasons for this is that your metabolism slows with age, so the amount of calories you need to survive even when resting drops by about 2 percent per decade throughout adulthood. If you don't cut back on your calorie intake, that metabolic slowdown can lead to a gain of two to three pounds per year—or twenty to thirty pounds per decade! Also, many transitional women are less active than they used to be, spending more time in their cars and less time walking than they used to. If you have a sedentary but time-consuming job or a life-style that doesn't leave you much time or energy to work out, your lack of exercise—coupled with your more sluggish metabolism—creates a perfect recipe for gaining more than a few unwanted pounds.

To keep your weight in the healthy range, you need to do a few things. One is to exercise. Not only will exercise spark your metabolism, but it also will:

- *Slow bone loss* and thus decrease your risk for osteoporosis.
- *Strengthen your heart and lungs.*
- *Improve your muscle tone.*
- *Increase your energy level.*
- *Help you manage the stress* so endemic to the transitional years.

If you can work thirty to sixty minutes of moderate aerobic exercise into your schedule at least three times a week (every day would be better, if you have the time), you'll stay more fit and keep your body humming along nicely throughout the transitional years. Activities such as walking, tennis, bicycling, and swimming improve your stamina by stimulating your nervous system to produce adrenaline, which increases your metabolism and vigor.

Just don't overdo it. An overly rigorous exercise regimen can change the way the brain controls the reproductive system, causing hormones to enter the bloodstream in smaller amounts than you need to function optimally. This can cause you to stop menstruating, at least temporarily. (Even if your menstrual cycles stay regular, overexercising can still weaken your fertility.) Female marathoners, for instance, often stop having periods because their long hours of training trigger an oversecretion of endorphins that inhibits hormone secretions from the pituitary gland. In turn, this reduces secretion of estrogen from the ovary. The resulting hormonal imbalance can cause their periods to stop or to occur irregularly.

Obviously, this is something you need to avoid if you're interested in staying fertile during your transitional years. Even if you don't want to get pregnant, it isn't a good idea to shut down your periods because the rapid reduction of estrogen can speed up bone loss and lead to premature osteoporosis.

In addition to exercising, maintaining your ideal weight involves eating a nutritionally dense diet. If you're constantly trying to shed a few pounds by skipping breakfast (triggering a mid-morning drop in blood sugar), taking in fewer than 1,200 calories a day, or existing on only one type of "healthy food" such as grapefruit or yogurt for more than a day or two, you may lose a few pounds temporarily (that is, until you go back to your old eating habits), but your body isn't going to get the nutrients it needs to keep your energy level up. The same is true if you're addicted to junk foods. Sorry—cookies, ice cream, potato chips, and chocolate do not make up the four food groups and they aren't going to keep your energy levels high. To maintain your stamina and your optimal weight, you need to get the most nutrition out of the 1,800 or so calories you take in every day by choosing a balanced mix of foods from the following four food groups:

- *Fruits and vegetables.* Eat two to four servings of fruit and three to five servings of vegetables daily. (A serving equals one medium piece of fruit or one half cup raw or cooked fruit or vegetables.) These choices should include foods high in vitamin C, including citrus fruits, melons, tomatoes, peppers, and cabbage; those high in vitamin A, including deep yellow and orange-colored vegetables and fruits such as winter squash, carrots, and apricots; and vegetables high in calcium, such as broccoli and kale.

• *Grains and cereals.* Eat six or more servings from this food group, with special emphasis on whole grains that contain trace minerals and fiber lacking in refined products. (One slice of bread, one ounce of cold cereal, or one half cup of cooked cereal, rice, or pasta is a serving.)

• *Milk and dairy products.* An excellent source of calcium; make sure you get two servings in your daily diet. (A serving is a cup of skim milk or yogurt, or one and a half ounces of natural cheese.) Choose skim milk, as well as low-fat or nonfat dairy products, to avoid excess fat.

• *Protein foods.* Americans tend to eat too much protein, so try to limit your intake to two three-ounce servings per day, or about five to seven ounces daily. And stick to lean meat, fish, or poultry (don't forget to remove the fatty skin on poultry); for vegetarians, one half cup cooked dried beans or peas equals an ounce of meat.

It's also smart to limit your consumption of fat, not only to keep your weight under control but also because fat has been linked with all sorts of ailments, including heart disease and certain cancers. Avoid sugar, too, mostly because it makes more fat. You need to limit your fat consumption to no more than 30 percent of daily calories.

If you eat a complete, well-balanced diet, you'll also get the beneficial effects of antioxidants. Antioxidants—including vitamins C, E, beta carotene (which the body turns into vitamin A), and selenium—are important because as we age our cells are increasingly damaged by a by-product of oxygen metabolism. Although our bodies need oxygen to live, the breakdown of oxygen as it passes through our cells results in substances called free radicals that attack and destroy membranes. The longer this happens, the less effectively our cells function. Antioxidants seem to combat the damaging effect of free radicals. And, as a growing body of research being done at Johns Hopkins University Medical Center and other medical facilities is beginning to reveal, this may help to ward off such serious illnesses as heart disease and cancer.

If you're not sure you're getting the optimum amount of vitamins and minerals, take a daily multivitamin. Just remember: if you eat a well-balanced diet, costly vitamin supplements aren't necessary.

7. *Quit smoking and avoid alcohol and caffeine.*

Despite all the warnings, nearly one third of women over thirty-five still smoke. If you're in this group, maybe this piece of information will get you to quit: women smokers tend to go through menopause five to ten years earlier than their nonsmoking relatives!

One possible reason is that nicotine may cause the ovaries to produce less estrogen. Another is that smoking may affect how the liver breaks down estrogen. Normally the liver detoxifies estrogen so that the kidneys can eliminate whatever isn't needed, but smoking interferes with this process, causing the liver to destroy too much of the most useful form of estrogen, leaving the body in short supply. If you *stop* smoking, though, your blood estrogen level can return to normal within three to four months.

If you want to stretch your fertile years, you need to quit smoking *now* in order to increase your chances of getting pregnant. Because tobacco smoke interferes with the implantation of a fertilized egg within the uterus and reduces the number of quality sperm cells in a man's ejaculate, couples in which at least one member smokes are much less likely to conceive than nonsmoking couples.

Transitional women interested in keeping midlife at bay also should steer clear of alcohol, or at least limit drinking to modest amounts—no more than two drinks a day. (A "drink" is three to five ounces of wine, twelve ounces of beer, or one ounce of hard liquor.) In addition to making your heart race and blood pressure climb, alcohol is toxic to your liver. If your liver can't function correctly, your body may be unable to properly regulate estrogen levels in the blood. This can lead to all the problems associated with inadequate estrogen levels—premature menopause, sagging breasts, dry skin and mucous membranes, and so on. Excessive alcohol has been known to cause irregular periods as well.

Caffeine is problematic for transitional women for several important reasons. For starters, preliminary research has linked it with an increased risk of uterine cancer. There is also evidence that caffeine can cause heavy menstrual bleeding and can inhibit ovulation. In addition, too much caffeine can make you overly tense before and during your periods. So be sure to limit coffee, tea, and caffeine-containing soft drinks such as colas to two or three cups per day. (Watch out for chocolate, too. It's got caffeine *and* fat.)

8. *Avoid unnecessary gynecological surgery.*

Eleanor, forty-three, recently came to me for a second opinion. She'd been diagnosed with a small uterine fibroid—less than an inch in size—and her doctor was insisting that she have a hysterectomy. But she was very reluctant to follow his advice.

"I'm really worried," she said. "A hysterectomy is such a drastic procedure. It's not that I want any more kids—three is plenty, believe me. But won't a hysterectomy make me menopausal . . . you know, hot flashes and all the rest? I don't want to be old before my time, so I guess my question is, is this absolutely necessary? Aren't there any other alternatives?"

Absolutely. While a hysterectomy is necessary for such problems as an excessively large fibroid or certain cancers, Eleanor was quite right in her belief that hysterectomy is major surgery and should not be undergone without full consideration of all the options. So she and I spent some time discussing them.

We talked about her taking medication, such as Lupron or Synerel, which could change her hormonal balance and help reduce the total size of the uterus, including the fibroid. We also discussed a hysteroscopy, a fairly simple procedure that can be used to remove a submucous fibroid, one located beneath the mucous membrane of the uterus. Another possibility is a myomectomy, a procedure used to remove a fibroid located on the outside of the uterus. (For more on these two procedures, see Chapter Six.) In Eleanor's case, another option was to do nothing. The fibroid was not causing her any serious symptoms, so we decided to wait and see if it grew large enough to be a problem.

Janet, forty, is another good example. When she complained of mid-cycle bleeding, her doctor insisted on a D&C (dilation and curettage, or scraping of the lining of the uterus) to discover what was wrong.

Janet was not aware that there are modern diagnostic tests that are much less invasive than a D&C. An endometrial sampling (also called an endometrial biopsy) is a simple office procedure that could have detected endometrial cancer or precancerous cell changes. During this procedure, a thin, plastic, strawlike tube is inserted into the uterus. Loose samples of the endometrium are sucked into it and sent to a lab to be analyzed. Another possible option might have been ultrasound, a completely noninvasive procedure that's very effective in diagnosing fibroids.

As it turned out, Janet had neither cancer nor fibroids, which these tests most likely would have revealed. In fact, Janet's D&C failed to uncover any medical problem that needed treatment.

As these two hypothetical stories illustrate, sometimes doctors recommend a surgical procedure, especially D&C or hysterectomy, without discussing possible alternatives with their patients. These procedures are often unnecessary or overly drastic, particularly for transitional women who would like to postpone menopause, who hope to stretch their reproductive years, or who may be concerned about the risks and stress of surgery. Remember, your body will not recuperate from such trauma as quickly as it did when you were younger. So be aware that you may have choices.

9. *Learn the newest methods for coping with stress.*

These days, stress seems to be part and parcel of the transitional years. Age-related changes such as wrinkles or "age spots" may depress you. Premenopausal symptoms such as irregular periods or hot flashes may make you feel anxious. Hormonal changes can heighten those feelings, especially around the time of your period. Add a hectic home life and/or a demanding career, and the stress on transitional women mounts. So if you're feeling more moody or irritable, join the crowd.

While you will feel better once you learn how to manage your physical problems, you probably won't be at your best until you also deal with the psychological side of the "body/mind" connection. Try the approaches to stress reduction, such as deep breathing, muscle relaxation, massage, guided imagery, and yoga, detailed in Chapter Twelve.

10. *Have noninvasive "wellness" tests.*

Even if you're feeling great, you'll need periodic medical checkups to screen for ailments common to the transitional years. The goal is to detect problems *before* you notice any symptoms so that you can maximize your chances of beating any disease.

Take breast cancer, for example. You know that if breast cancer is detected early, the chances of effective yet less destructive treatment, such as a lumpectomy instead of a mastectomy, increase enormously. And to date, the best way to detect any problems is to do a breast self-examination once a month in conjunction with having your doctor perform a physical examination of your breasts at least once a year. Approximately 70 to 75 percent of all breast cancers are detected by these exams alone. And despite the fact that the benefit of mammograms for women under age fifty has recently been called into question, statistics still tell a different story. Statistically, 80 to 85 percent of breast cancers are detected when mammograms are done in addition to regular physical breast exams.

The American Cancer Society still recommends that every woman get an initial mammogram somewhere between ages thirty-five and forty, then another every eighteen to twenty-four months through her forties, with yearly mammograms after age fifty.

I've created a helpful chart at the end of this book (see Appendix B) showing which tests I feel are very important, as well as when and how often you should have them. But let me stress now that you should have periodic blood pressure and cholesterol tests, Pap smears, mammograms, stool and rectal exams, and dental checkups. How often you have these tests performed depends on your age and the kind of results you get. The need for other screenings, such as the

Natural Ways to Maximize Your Vitality

TSH (thyroid) test or electrocardiograms, depends upon your symptoms and medical history.

Learning to outsmart many of the problems common to the transitional years isn't all that difficult, but you need to take responsibility for your body and stick to these well-tested guidelines. You may need to make life-style changes, and you may need to be receptive to certain tests and treatments while working with your doctor to decide whether they're right for you, with your unique body type, health history, daily routine, and goals. Most importantly, you need to remind yourself that you're a valuable, vital individual whose best is yet to come!

3

Coping with Menstrual Changes

- Menstrual Changes You May Experience
- Simple and Sound Ways to Alleviate Troublesome Symptoms
- Should You Start Taking the Pill?
- Understanding Progesterone Therapy
- Is Estrogen for You?
- Real Women, Real Problems—Real Remedies

At about age thirty-six, the very start of your transitional years, your menstrual cycles begin to change. Early on, these changes are usually minor, perhaps an occasionally longer or shorter period with slightly heavier or lighter flow. Such early changes rarely cause any discomfort or disruption in your day-to-day routine. In fact, these menstrual shifts can be so subtle that you might not even notice them.

But as you get older, changes in your periods often become too frequent or dramatic to ignore. You may find that you're bleeding much more heavily (menorrhagia) or for an unusually long time (hypermenorrhea), or that your period now comes and goes within seventy-two hours (hypomenorrhea). You may start getting periods that flip-flop from heavy to light to heavy again—although about 50 percent of women change in one direction or the other—or you may even miss a period or two.

Because these changes are such a departure from the menstrual pattern you've known for so many years, they can be pretty scary. Many of my patients become alarmed, wondering if something is seriously wrong with them.

Usually these changes aren't anything to worry about. Most often, they're the result of the normal premenopausal hormonal shifts that mark the transitional years in many healthy women.

With age, the ovarian and pituitary hormones that so effectively controlled your monthly cycle when you were younger don't do their job as well as they once did. The result is increasingly irregular, sometimes messy, and possibly painful menstrual periods.

Although menstrual changes are natural, they can still be hard on your body. Every menstrual bleed consists of both blood and endometrial tissue: the blood is shed when a blood vessel that supplies this area of the endometrium breaks off during menstruation; the endometrial tissue comes from the sloughing off of the uterine lining. You lose approximately fifty to seventy-five milliliters of blood in a normal period. But excessive menstrual bleeding—a loss of eighty or more milliliters—even during a single period, can lower your hemoglobin (the iron-containing portion of your red blood cells) enough to make you feel tired and washed out.

Normally, your spleen and bone marrow work harder for a few days each month in order to put out more platelets, which replenish red blood cells lost during menstruation.

When you get a heavy loss each month, however, your body cannot replace these cells fast enough and you can become anemic.

In some cases, menstrual changes can be a sign of an underlying medical problem. A bout of mid-cycle spotting, for example, could signal a problem such as fibroids, or even cancer.

If your periods have become troublesome, take heart. As long as you are otherwise healthy, you'll probably be able to feel comfortable again. Today's excellent treatment options, ranging from diet and exercise to birth control pills and even estrogen therapy, can end or at least minimize any bothersome menstrual changes and, while they're at it, delay early menopausal symptoms or eliminate them forever.

Menstrual Changes You May Experience

No one can predict exactly how your menstrual cycles will change during your transitional years. Every woman's body behaves differently. Because your hormones start to decrease both in amount and effectiveness after age thirty-six, one or more problems typically appear:

An unusually heavy menstrual bleed.

If you think back to what you learned in school about biology and human reproduction (remember Biology 101?), you'll recall that at a certain point in your cycle, your ovaries begin to secrete estrogen. This causes the lining of your uterus, or the endometrium, to increase in size, first by thickening its "basalis" layer, by increasing both the number and the size of cells, and then, as estrogen keeps building, by causing a spongy, soft layer called the "spongiosa" to grow on top of it. After ovulation, when both estrogen and progesterone are released into the bloodstream, a third layer, called the "compacta," begins to grow. This layer compacts the layers of the endometrium and prepares them to receive and protect the fertilized egg should pregnancy occur.

A small bump called the "corpus luteum" is formed on the ovary at the place where the dominant follicle ruptured as it thrust its egg out toward the fallopian tubes. The corpus luteum secretes both estrogen and progesterone. If pregnancy does not occur, the corpus luteum degenerates in the ovary about two weeks after you ovulate. Hormone levels decrease and the top two layers of the endometrium are sloughed off in what we know as normal menstruation. (For a quick refresher course in the female reproductive cycle, see Appendix A.)

Now if you don't have enough estrogen, you don't ovulate and there's no corpus luteum to secrete progesterone—thus, you do not have a menstrual cycle. Without the right amount of estrogen and with no progesterone, you don't get any compacta layer, either; instead, the spongiosa grows unchecked until it becomes so heavy that it breaks away from the remaining basalis layer of the endometrium and flows away in a bright red, clotty, and unusually heavy menstrual bleed, known as "breakthrough bleeding." Since there is no cycle, breakthrough bleeding can occur at any time.

Variable bleeding.

In a younger woman, the uterus responds evenly to circulating estrogen, so that when it sheds its endometrium during menstruation, the layers fall off in a continuous way, causing a fairly steady menstrual flow. But in your transitional years, hormonal shifts can cause the endometrium to respond in an uneven manner. Parts of it are sloughed off at certain times, other parts at other times. Thus, heavy bleeding occurs as one section of the endometrium sheds, followed by a slight bleed as a little from another part sheds, then a heavy bleed as a third part falls away. Think of it as you would different sections of a flower bed: some bloom first, then begin to fade just as others start blossoming.

"Early" bleeding or menstrual spotting.

Again, let's flash back to Biology 101. You'll recall that during the normal reproductive cycle, estrogen levels continue to build until there is sufficient estrogen in the blood to telegraph to the pituitary gland that it is time to release a surge of luteinizing hormone (LH), which brings about ovulation. But if estrogen levels never get high enough and instead plateau before they can trigger the pituitary to release the LH surge—and if estrogen then dips below a certain threshold—the endometrium will be sloughed off from the inside of the uterus before it has a chance to grow very much. Ovulation does not occur, and therefore your usual menstrual cycle does not occur either. What does transpire is a minimal bleed called "withdrawal bleeding" that could start any time in your cycle, often earlier than you expect to bleed, and that can last for several days.

Shorter periods with less flow—or no period at all.

If your estrogen levels are low, your uterus will grow only a very thin endometrial lining during the monthly cycle. When this happens, you may slough off that lining in an unusually shorter or lighter menstrual period.

If the lining is so insufficient that there is literally nothing to slough off, you may not have any menses at all. When this happens for a period or two, it's called "oligomenorrhea." If you don't get your period for more than three months, it's called "amenorrhea," which simply means the absence of any menstrual bleeding. Both oligomenorrhea and amenorrhea can be caused by lack of ovulation and/or too little estrogen.

Persistent spotting.

Occasionally you may "spot" just before or after you have your period; you'll see a pinkish to dark bloodstain on your clothing or pantyliners. No one really knows why premenstrual spotting occurs, although we believe it's caused by some uneven shedding of the endometrium. Dark spotting *after* your period is sometimes the result of blood that was retained in the uterus or the vagina and that trickles out later. Either kind of spotting, as long as it occurs immediately around the time of your period, is usually harmless and needs no treatment.

Mid-cycle spotting.

Of all the menstrual changes you may encounter, the one that should always put you on alert is mid-cycle or "intracycle" spotting. Lots of times, it's nothing more than *Mittelschmerz* (German for "middle of the period"), harmless bleeding that occurs when you ovulate and blood from the ruptured follicle finds its way through the fallopian tube, through the cervix, and out the vagina.

Mid-cycle spotting, however, can be a symptom of cancer of the endometrium (uterine cancer). The big problem is that there's no way to tell without running a few tests, including an endometrial biopsy, a simple office procedure in which a sample is taken from the inside of the uterus. If the results of this preliminary test suggest a problem, your doctor will want to do a D&C to get more information.

Before you start biting your nails, though, let me add a qualifier here. If over the years you've frequently spotted at mid-cycle and you've never had any problems, such spotting during your transitional years is probably normal for you. Even if it has never happened to you before, it doesn't necessarily mean you've got cancer. So don't panic. Approximately 95 percent of endometrial samples turn out to be benign. But since mid-cycle spotting *could* be caused by cancer, as well as by fibroids, miscarriage, or ectopic pregnancy, it's always best to work with your doctor to determine the underlying problem.

Simple and Sound Ways to Alleviate Troublesome Symptoms

Most transitional women will experience at least one of the menstrual changes we've just discussed. As long as the changes in your cycle don't threaten your health or well-being—for example, very heavy bleeding could cause you to become anemic, or failing to ovulate could keep you from becoming pregnant—you may decide you don't need to do anything about them. But I believe that if these menstrual shifts are bothersome at all—for example, if unexpected bleeding catches you unprepared and causes you embarrassment, or if clotting leads to cramping or backaches—you can and should seek out the right remedies. Here are today's most effective options, starting with simple and sound approaches to overall healthy living.

Just the right exercise.

As I explained in the previous chapter, too much exercise can make you stop menstruating. This complicates the hormonal picture for transitional women. If you already have skipped a period or two and are involved in a demanding exercise program, cutting back a bit may help your menses return.

On the other hand, sedentary women, particularly when they are under stress, tend to experience more menstrual irregularities than women who exercise on a routine basis. Many patients have told me that their periods become more irregular and that their flow either intensifies or decreases when they're not only under a great deal of emotional and psychological strain but also are physically inactive.

If the changes in your period are fairly mild but still annoying enough for you to want to alleviate them, try maintaining a sound, regular exercise program consisting of about thirty to sixty minutes of moderate aerobic exercise at least three times a week. Walking, swimming, bicycling, jogging, and aerobic dancing are good choices. As long as you clear it with your physician, such a program won't hurt—and may help you ease your menstrual problems and maintain a better level of overall fitness and health.

Everybody needs exercise, and the benefits of a regular workout go beyond menstrual regularity. Before you think about taking medication to alleviate your premenopausal symptoms, see if simply exercising is helpful. Even if you ultimately end up treating your problem with medication, the exercise will continue to bring you health benefits that no prescription can provide.

Smart eating.

As I already mentioned in my Ten-Point Plan for Peak Health and Vitality, being too fat or too thin can provoke many of the menstrual irregularities we've just discussed. This means weight control is more than just a cosmetic issue for transitional women. "Smart eating" means choosing healthful foods and, as I mentioned earlier, avoiding fat, sugar, alcohol, and caffeine. Overdosing on salt can contribute to premenstrual bloating, so steer clear of those nachos when that little voice inside you urges you to have "just one."

Home remedies.

If you're into home treatments, here are a few that may help straighten out your menstrual problems:

- Foods high in vitamin C may help with heavy or irregular bleeding. The theory is that because it's an antioxidant, vitamin C could help counteract the effect of too many free radicals that may impair normal menstrual functioning.
- Heavy bleeding has been linked with a deficiency of vitamin A. So if this is your problem, try eating foods packed with carotene (including carrots, kale, spinach, sweet potatoes, and winter squash).
- Raspberry or camomile tea may ease the cramping that often accompanies heavy menstrual bleeding.
- Some say pennyroyal leaf tea (*not* the toxic oil) helps alleviate a lack of menstrual flow. But do be sure to limit your consumption to one or two cups a day, and use this with caution.

Since I don't know of any definitive studies that support these claims, I can't recommend home remedies in place of more scientifically tested remedies. On the other hand, if done in moderation, they can't hurt, so if you want to give them a try, go ahead. Just be sure to check with your doctor first to see if he or she raises any objections.

Good sex.

As I mentioned in the last chapter, an active sex life helps maintain high estrogen levels, which can have a beneficial effect on your periods. We really don't understand why any regular sexual activity—not only intercourse, but kissing, petting, or any other activity that gets you stimulated—seems helpful, but it probably has something to do with keeping your sexual organs in good working order. So if you're in the mood, go for it!

If life-style changes—eating right, exercising, reducing stress, and enjoying sexual relations when possible—don't alleviate your menstrual troubles, it may be time to consider hormonal treatments. You may have more options with this approach than you realize.

Estrogen is vital to a woman's overall health and well-being. That's why for years doctors have prescribed estrogen replacement therapy (ERT) for menopausal women whose estrogen levels have plummeted. Today, however, more gynecologists and reproductive endocrinologists like myself are finding that estrogen and other hormones can help transitional women, too.

Estrogen is not a panacea for every problem or individual, and it does have the potential for some serious side effects, which I'll discuss later. Nonetheless, I find that in many cases the possible benefits of estrogen can outweigh the risks, making estrogen therapy worth considering.

Should You Start Taking the Pill?

While you may not consider birth control pills (also known as BCP or the Pill) a form of hormone replacement therapy, that's exactly what they are. BCP generally consists of combinations of different doses of estrogen, or ethinyl estradiol, and progestins, steroid hormones that act like the natural hormone progesterone, which play a key role in regulating your cycle.

I prescribe birth control pills to transitional women for two main reasons. First, they do an excellent job of regulating your cycle so that your periods appear at evenly timed, regular intervals. Second, by making sure the endometrium is getting enough estrogen and progesterone, they protect the overall health of the uterus. BCP also helps prevent the formation of hormonal cysts on the ovaries. (Although these cysts are benign, they can be extremely painful, even to the point of requiring ovarian surgery, which can cause some menopausal symptoms.) Of course, BCP also offers nearly foolproof protection against unwanted pregnancy, another benefit not to be overlooked in the transitional years.

Birth control pills are given in packs of twenty-one or twenty-eight. After twenty-one days of hormone therapy, you take a break for a week (which is when you get your period). A twenty-eight-pack contains seven placebo pills so you can take a pill each day and not worry about what day it is.

If you're suffering from an acute problem such as sudden and very intense menstrual bleeding, most doctors will treat it with birth control pills but use them a little differently. They'll divide a pack of BCP and advise you to take three daily for seven days so that the excessive bleeding will stop. If your cycles then revert to normal in the months that follow, there's no reason for you to continue taking the Pill. But if you're bothered by a persistent problem, you can safely take BCP in the usual manner for as long as you like.

You may be surprised to find me recommending the Pill to transitional women. Until fairly recently, doctors limited use of the Pill to women under the age of thirty-five because as women move beyond that age they are at increasingly higher risk for potential side effects, such as stroke and blood clots. But in the past decade or so, new formulations of BCP containing far lower hormone dosages have become available (thirty-five micrograms of estrogen as opposed to fifty). They've sharply reduced the incidence of side effects, making the Pill safe for many healthy women over thirty-five. In fact, in 1990, the U.S. Food and Drug Administration's advisory committee voted to change the product labeling on the Pill to allow doctors to prescribe BCP to healthy non-smoking women over thirty-five.

(FYI: An extremely low dosage BCP containing twenty to twenty-five micrograms of estrogen is now on the market, which should provide an additional margin of safety for transitional women, although we will have to wait for more data to be available to know definitely if this dosage lowers risk even more significantly without losing effectiveness.)

The downside of the pill.

As wonderfully effective as the Pill is in treating menstrual problems, it does have its drawbacks. Some women experience two to three months of breakthrough bleeding because the persistent levels of estrogen that they are taking with the Pill cannot initially maintain the lining of the endometrium. If this occurs, tell your doctor. He or she may want to give you some additional estrogen for a few months, or may recommend that you switch to another brand of BCP that may work better. An initial problem does not necessarily rule out BCP for you; your body may just need time to adjust. If problems persist for more than three months, you may just need a different formulation.

One of the most serious side effects of taking oral contraceptives is the risk of developing blood clots. These clots can cause serious problems such as thrombophlebitis (an inflammation of the veins of the leg), cardiac disease, pulmonary difficulties, stroke, and in some cases even death. Understand, however, that these risks are mostly associated with higher dosage pills than those we now prescribe. Also, the problem is rare; in women twenty to forty-four, about one in two thousand will be hospitalized each year because of abnormal clotting. And the risk of death due to circulatory problems associated with higher dosage pills is even lower.

BCP users may have a slightly greater risk than nonusers of having gallbladder problems, although this risk is probably related to high-dose estrogen pills that are no longer prescribed. In *very* rare cases, BCP may also cause benign liver tumors, although no definite association between the Pill and these tumors has been found.

Sometimes women fear that they'll become so dependent on BCP that they'll never be able to stop taking it. In my thirty-plus years of practice, I've never seen this happen. The Pill is not addictive. Your body does get used to the daily dose of hormones, but you don't need the Pill to keep functioning. I've had hundreds of patients take BCP for months, and even years, then stop at will.

The pill and cancer.

Again and again, I find that transitional women are reluctant to go on BCP for fear that they may be putting themselves at greater risk for cancer. They are wise to be cautious, but the pill has come a long way in twenty years.

Back in the seventies, studies showed that women on BCP had higher incidence of certain types of cancers, including cancer of the uterus and breast. But these early pills contained much higher doses of estrogen—as much as 180 micrograms as opposed to today's 20-to-35-microgram doses. More recent studies show that the Pill cuts in half the risk of endometrial cancer if a woman takes it for at least four years.

Controversy still surrounds the issue of whether or not BCP increases a woman's risk for breast cancer. However, in the September 1992 issue of *Obstetrics and Gynecology*, a review of the major research studies on BCP and breast cancer concludes that, with few exceptions, neither birth control pills nor estrogen therapy have been shown to raise the risk of breast cancer. The exceptions involve women who have taken high doses of estrogen or high-dose BCP for several years. Still, if you are already at high risk for breast cancer—for instance, if your mother or sister had the disease—you want to be very cautious about taking BCP—or estrogen, for that matter. High-risk women should talk with their doctors at length about the best course of treatment for them. (For more information about estrogen, BCP, and cancer, see Chapter Ten.)

Information on BCP and ovarian cancer is a lot more clear and encouraging. Several studies, including a 1987 study from the Centers for Disease Control, has shown that women who take today's Pill, even if only for a few months, have a forty percent *lower* chance of developing the most common form of ovarian cancer. This protective benefit lasts many years after you stop using the Pill.

You don't have to worry about BCP increasing your risk for uterine cancer, either. As long as the Pill contains a combination of estrogen and progesterone—and all of today's birth control pills do—you're at no greater risk for uterine cancer than women not on the Pill.

Who should not take the pill.

Though BCP is highly effective and safe for most women, taking it shouldn't be a casual decision. If you're over thirty-five, you should be carefully screened by your doctor to make sure the Pill is right for you. That is, your doctor would make sure that your Pap test is clear, that you don't have any masses in the pelvic or abdominal area, and that you have no history of heart attack, stroke, blood clots, or high blood pressure.

- *Don't take the Pill if you have or have ever had breast cancer,* particularly if that cancer was estrogen dependent. Going on the Pill could increase your risk that the cancer will recur.
- *The Pill can complicate existing medical conditions.* Don't take the Pill if you have chest pain, a history of heart attack, stroke, blood clots, or liver tumors (either benign or malignant).
- *Don't take the Pill if you could be pregnant.*
- *Women who smoke should stay away from BCP.* Smoking is associated with higher risk for cardiac, vascular, pulmonary, and liver problems that birth control pills could exacerbate. The good news is that if you stop smoking for at least one year, you can take the Pill without any increased risk.

Guidelines for taking the pill.

If you do choose BCP, follow these guidelines to maximize the benefits and minimize any side effects.

• *Ask your doctor to prescribe the BCP with the lowest possible amount of estrogen and progesterone effective for you.* There aren't any tests that can identify the lowest effective formulation or dosage for you; a lot depends upon your age, previous history with BCP, and your goal in taking it (that is, whether to regulate your period, have a lighter period, or whatever). It's best to start with the lowest dosage available and see if that solves the problem; if not, dosages should be built up slowly until the optimal is reached. But as I've explained earlier, transitional women should avoid using any pill that contains more than thirty-five micrograms of ethinyl estradiol (active estrogen).

• *See your gynecologist at least annually—and preferably every six months—for a checkup.*

• *Make sure you perform monthly breast self-exams and get regular mammograms.*

• *Let your doctor know if you notice any vaginal bleeding or spotting between periods.* Although spotting is a common side effect among new Pill users and usually goes away within a few months, if the problem persists your doctor may want to perform some of the tests we've already discussed.

UNDERSTANDING PROGESTERONE THERAPY

Another way to ease your menstrual problems, particularly those that may occur when you don't ovulate, is progesterone therapy. By getting an injection of progesterone or taking oral progestins (synthetic drugs that have a progesterone-like effect on the body) during the second half of your cycle—the point at which, after ovulation in a normal cycle, your own progesterone would kick in—you can improve overly light or missing periods. Surprisingly, progesterone can also help alleviate heavy periods.

Here's why. If your period is light or missing, it means your endometrium is growing unchecked; eventually, it will grow so much that you will start bleeding, and probably very heavily. Since progesterone allows the final layer, the compacta, of your endometrium to form—thus preventing the endometrium from growing unchecked—progesterone therapy can regulate your periods so that they are neither overly light nor missing. This therapy can also eliminate or reduce any breakthrough bleeding.

Progesterone or progestin therapy has an additional benefit: it may help prevent endometrial cancer. Again, the reason is that if you don't have progesterone, your endometrium may start to overgrow (a condition known as endometrial hyperplasia), setting the stage for premalignant changes. But progesterone helps form the compact layer, which, in turn, acts on the endometrium to help prepare it for pregnancy, or, if no pregnancy occurs, for a clean break from the basalis layer of the uterus. In the absence of naturally secreted progesterone, progesterone therapy does the same thing, thus reducing the risk of endometrial hyperplasia and cancer.

The most widely prescribed oral progestin is medroxyprogesterone acetate (MPA), which you may know by its brand names, Provera or Cycrin. Generally, MPA is given for five to ten days a month, although most commonly on days twenty to twenty-four from the first day of your period (for ten-day dosages, you would start on day fifteen). I usually prescribe a dose that ranges from two and a half milligrams to ten milligrams a day. (Some doctors prefer the progestins Norlutate or megestrol, since they believe these medications *may* help prevent cholesterol levels from rising. But these medications can cause undesirable side effects, such as oily skin and the growth of unwanted facial and body hair, so I don't like to use them.)

Most women find relief with progesterone therapy quickly, either getting a period within ten days or experiencing much less breakthrough bleeding. After one or two months of therapy, you have three options:

1. Stop taking the progesterone and see if your body regulates itself.
2. Continue with progesterone for a few more months and then see how you do on your own.
3. Stop the progestrone and start taking birth control pills.

Women who have not been ovulating and who start progesterone therapy may start ovulating again, which makes pregnancy a possibility. Some women are thrilled about this and some aren't. If you don't want to get pregnant, be sure to review your birth control options with your doctor.

Though highly effective, progesterone therapy isn't perfect. It may cause you to suffer such side effects as breast tenderness, irritability, abdominal bloating, occasional nausea, insomnia, or even a slight increase in hairiness. Sometimes you can find relief by switching to another type of progesterone or asking your doctor to make a small downward adjustment in the hormone dose.

Another possible drawback: progesterone may cause a mild increase in your cholesterol levels. This is not a major problem, however, because you are taking progesterone for only a few days per month; when you stop taking it, cholesterol levels return to the levels usual for you.

Is Estrogen for You?

If you're suffering from a combination of complaints—for example, menstrual irregularities accompanied by such estrogen-deprivation symptoms as hot flashes, heightened PMS, or reduced vaginal secretions—and you haven't had any success alleviating your problems with exercise, diet, home remedies, or alternative remedies such as acupuncture or yoga, you're an excellent candidate for estrogen therapy.

Let me say right up front that this is a relatively new type of therapy for women in your age group and an approach that up until recently raised more than a few eyebrows. That's because for years it was assumed that only menopausal women had severe enough estrogen deficits to benefit from supplemental estrogen. In the late 1980s, however, researchers, myself among them, revealed the results of some pioneering studies that finally challenged that assumption. A study my research group conducted at the Medical College of Pennsylvania in 1988 showed that premenopausal, transitional women as young as thirty-five can also suffer from insufficient estrogen and, therefore, can enjoy the benefits of very low doses of estrogen.

When I have a patient whose particular mix of menstrual problems and estrogen-deprivation symptoms makes her a prime candidate for estrogen supplement therapy (EST), I usually prescribe small amounts of estrogen for the first ten days of her cycle. In case after case, I've found that after about six months, estrogen levels build up enough not only to bring about a more normal, comfortable menstrual period but also to ease other estrogen-related problems as well. After six months, we are usually able to scale back the dosage to a minimal level or to discontinue treatment altogether.

Estrogen supplement therapy is not to be confused with traditional estrogen replacement therapy (ERT). The supplemental approach uses a smaller dosage of estrogen, just enough to spark your body to produce its own progesterone, which in turn naturally protects the uterus from cancer and helps restore a normal, healthy menstrual period.

If supplemental estrogen alone doesn't do the trick, ask your doctor about *cyclic therapy*. With cyclic therapy, you take estrogen alone for nineteen days, after which you take a combination of estrogen and progesterone (or progestin) for the last five or so days. The hope is that after a few months these added hormones will jump start your pituitary gland to release other hormones that, in turn, stimulate the ovaries to release sufficient amounts of estrogen and progesterone without any outside help. At that point, you'll be able to stop taking any medication and function normally on your own.

Who should not have estrogen therapy.

If you've ever been bothered by any heart or circulation problems, including high blood pressure, abnormal blood clotting, or stroke, estrogen therapy is probably not for you. It is also not appropriate or recommended for women who smoke or have had a liver tumor, or who are pregnant or have ever had cancer.

Guidelines for successful estrogen supplement therapy.

Your doctor will probably monitor your response to EST closely for the first six months. After that, you should see your doctor at least once a year, and inform him or her immediately if you notice any of these *rare* complications:

- *Abnormal vaginal bleeding,* which could signal an infection or a benign or malignant tumor of the uterus.
- *Calf or chest pains, sudden shortness of breath, or coughing up blood,* any of which could signal a blood clot in the upper body. (Estrogen has a tendency to increase certain clotting mechanisms in the blood.)
- *Severe headaches, dizziness, or faintness, or changes in vision,* which could signal a blood clot in your brain or eye.
- *Yellowing of your skin,* which might mean a liver problem.
- *Pain, swelling, or tenderness in your abdomen,* which could indicate a problem with your liver, gallbladder or gastrointestinal tract.

After learning about the benefits of estrogen therapy, some patients have raised these two important questions:

1. If hormones are so terrific, why do we ever have to go through menopause?
2. Can you restore your menstrual cycle forever?

When you take estrogen, you are directly affecting the endometrial lining, which has estrogen receptors, components in cells that combine with estrogen to alter the function of the cell. The lining will keep building up and sloughing off and you can get a period for many years, as long as you continue to take estrogen. As you age, however, the number of receptors that you form continues to decrease, despite the additional estrogen. Once the number of receptors gets very low, you will stop bleeding altogether, although that may not occur until your mid-seventies *if* you keep taking estrogen that long.

But even women who continue to bleed are not having a true menstrual or ovulatory period because the estrogen taken in hormone therapy does not restart ovarian function. Your ovaries quit at around fifty, the average age of menopause, no matter what. That means that after menopause, no eggs are being released and you are no longer fertile.

Real Women, Real Problems — Real Remedies

Now that you have a better idea of the menstrual changes transitional women can encounter, and of the newest and most effective ways to treat them, meet a few real-life women who've experienced both.

Betsy's odd period.

After having perfectly regular, predictable cycles for years, thirty-seven-year-old Betsy suddenly had a period in which she bled heavily for two days, spotted for the next two, then bled so heavily for two more days that she had to change her tampons every hour and wear pads to give herself additional protection. She also felt dizzy and weak. Then the bleeding suddenly stopped.

A pelvic exam revealed no medical problems and Betsy didn't have any other complaints, so I asked her to keep a diary over the next few months to see whether this odd period was a one-time occurrence or the beginning of a new menstrual pattern. After three months, it was clear that it had become a pattern. Because Betsy had always been in perfect health, I felt that this new pattern almost certainly was being triggered by a change in how her hormones were interacting. This, in turn, was causing irregular shedding of her endometrium.

This kind of menstrual change wasn't harmful to Betsy and didn't demand treatment; there was even the possibility that in time it would clear up on its own. But Betsy was troubled by the excessive bleeding and weakness that disrupted her life enough to cause her to miss a few days of work, something she couldn't afford in her high-pressured position as an insurance agent. So we discussed several possible options.

One was birth control pills. They would help Betsy maintain a constant hormonal environment in her uterus and endometrium, which, in turn, would give her a steady, predictable menstrual flow. Another choice was taking progesterone to normalize the lining of the endometrium and produce a more regular period. Or, if that tactic failed, she could try cyclic therapy with both estrogen and progesterone in a sequence similar to the normal cycle.

After much consideration, Betsy chose birth control pills because she wanted to be taking something that not only alleviated the problem but provided her with contraception, which she felt was also important. Her cycle is more regular and she's much more comfortable. Because she doesn't like the idea of being on pills for too long, she's planning to stop after about a year, at which time we will reevaluate her condition and decide whether or not she needs or wants further treatment.

Liz's period dragged on and on.

Liz, forty-two, came to me when her periods suddenly became quite heavy and lasted several days longer than usual. Her physical exam revealed no medical problems, so I asked Liz to keep track of the number of tampons she was using each day to help me gauge just how heavy her flow had been.

Because Liz told me that her flow had been quite heavy for her last three periods, I took a blood count to see if she had become anemic. First, I checked to make sure she was in the middle of her cycle. It's not a good idea to get a blood count right after your period—even a normal period—because you may show a misleadingly low count. For better accuracy, wait a few days instead.

Liz's blood tests revealed she was slightly anemic, so I recommended some long-acting iron pills for her to take daily. I usually suggest ferrous gluconate in time-release capsules or tablets—you can get these over the counter—because they allow the iron to go into the body very slowly, thereby preventing gastrointestinal upset.

Further tests ruled out tumors or miscarriage as the cause of Liz's persistent periods, so I was pretty certain her trouble was hormonal. First, I prescribed daily doses of progesterone for seven days to bring her menses under control. After that, Liz went on her present monthly treatment schedule of five days of progesterone (days twenty to twenty-four, counting from the first day of her period) for three months, after which I will reevaluate her to see if the medication can be stopped. I also reminded Liz that her fertility might be enhanced and that if she didn't want to become pregnant she must continue using her diaphragm and jelly.

Janice had all the usual premenstrual symptoms, but her period never came.

Janice, forty-two, a married woman with three children, was clearly worried. "My period never came, even though I had all the usual warning signs, and the results of my home pregnancy test just weren't clear. Do you think I could be pregnant again? Or is something wrong with me?"

We ran another pregnancy test, and the results were negative. A pelvic examination didn't reveal anything unusual, either. I knew that Janice had taken birth control pills until one year earlier, when she had decided to change her form of contraception to a diaphragm and jelly. While it is often true that immediately after stopping the Pill you may not become regular for a few cycles, I also knew that Janice's normal cycles had resumed.

As we talked, I learned that Janice had felt the usual premenstrual symptoms—breast tenderness, bloating, some mood swings—and that they had subsided, although her period had never come. Thus I thought the reason she hadn't menstruated was that she hadn't ovulated; that is, since she had neither breakthrough nor withdrawal bleeding, her estrogen levels either never got high enough or had fallen prematurely during her cycle, either of which would prevent ovulation from occurring.

Janice didn't want to have any more kids, so she wasn't worried about maintaining her fertility. When I assured Janice that an occasional missing period would not put her in any danger, she decided against any form of treatment. She did agree, however, to modify her diet by cutting down caffeine and salt to soothe some of her premenstrual symptoms.

Six months later, she was back. "Cutting down on caffeine did help with my breast tenderness and anxiety, no question," she said. "But now I've missed my period for three months, and I also think I had my first hot flash!"

This time around, Janice wanted to try treatment. So I offered her a choice: she could try taking progesterone to see if we could bring on a period, which would occur if she was producing enough estrogen on her own. Or she could get started on very low doses of estrogen, which might induce her to ovulate and secrete progesterone, thereby bringing on a period. Janice chose estrogen therapy because that approach made any future hot flashes extremely unlikely. Two years later, she's still taking estrogen and doing just fine.

Kathryn had no period for four months.

One day several years ago, Kathryn, forty-seven, was upset when she came to see me. "Bernie, you've got to help me. I haven't had a period in four months! I know I'm not pregnant. I guess it could be menopause, but aren't I too young yet? I'm not even fifty! Is this old age—or something horrible? Either option looks bad to me."

Since Kathryn was close to menopause, the first step was to test her FSH level. (Remember, FSH is one of two pituitary hormones—the other being luteinizing hormone, or LH—that control the activities of the ovaries. And a woman moving into menopause will experience a rise in FSH.) Sure enough, Kathryn's FSH was quite elevated, leading me to believe that her ovaries were no longer fully functioning and were not putting out adequate estrogen to cause cycles. (A rise in LH would indicate that the condition is much more advanced; that is, that the ovaries are almost completely inactive. But this was not the case with Kathryn.)

Before I could identify the best treatment for Kathryn, I had to answer one key question: did she have any estrogen at all? To find out, I prescribed progesterone (taken for five days); if Kathryn was still producing estrogen, she would have a withdrawal bleed from the endometrium—ranging from a drop or two of blood to a full menstrual bleed—within a few days after she stopped taking the progesterone. If nothing occurred, I'd be able to conclude that she had little to no estrogen—which is precisely what was happening in Kathryn's case.

To confirm further my belief that Kathryn lacked estrogen, I evaluated her for any other estrogen-deprivation problems and found she had several, including a dry vagina, loss of sexual interest, mood swings, and the growth of some facial hair. That's when it became crystal clear that Kathryn was heading into menopause and might do quite well with regular estrogen replacement therapy (ERT). Since there was nothing in her medical history that led me to believe ERT was inadvisable, I recommended treatment.

Kathryn began a program in which she took very low doses of estrogen for twenty-five days, the last ten days of which she also took progesterone. She got her period and she felt terrific. If Kathryn continues her treatment, which I recommend that she do, the hormonal therapy will allow her to move into menopause without any discomfort whatsoever.

Suzannah's mid-cycle spotting.

Forty-year-old Suzannah noticed some spotting about two weeks before her regular period was due. She knew this might signal a serious problem, so she came to see me immediately. I did a Pap smear to see if there was any malignancy in the cervix or the endocervix (the lining of the canal of the neck of the uterus). Happily, her Pap results were normal.

After Suzannah's spotting reappeared the following month,

I took an endometrial sampling to check for cancer or a tumor in her uterus. Because there were areas in the sample that were suspicious, I recommended that Suzannah undergo a fractional D&C, also known as an endocervical and endometrial curettage. This procedure, which requires general anesthesia and is more extensive than a regular D&C, is a thorough test for cancer because it examines tissue from both the endocervix and the endometrium. (In a regular D&C, material is taken only from the endometrium.)

The pathology report brought good news: Suzannah did not have cancer. Instead, her problem was hyperplasia of the endometrium, a buildup of cells that occurs when the estrogen levels do not get high enough to bring about ovulation. The sheer mass of the endometrium was causing Suzannah's mid-cycle bleeding. To treat this condition, Suzannah had two options: she could take progesterone for a few months in order to make her periods more predictable and regular, or could just live with it and wear a panty shield to avoid staining her clothing with any unexpected bleeding. Suzannah chose the latter, but is monitoring her situation closely. If she continues to stain for one year, I will recommend we do another office endometrial biopsy to see if there is any problematic change in the endometrial lining.

As you can see, while a host of menstrual changes and problems can pop up during the transitional years, there's often no reason for you to suffer, especially since so many excellent and safe remedies are available. The trick lies in knowing your body well enough to be able to spot any significant changes, and then bringing them to the attention of a doctor skilled in today's newest and most effective treatments.

4

Hot Flashes... At Your Age?

- Who Gets Hot Flashes?
- What Are Hot Flashes?
- How Many Hot Flashes Will You Have?
- What Causes Hot Flashes?
- Simple Treatments for Hot Flashes
- Hormone Replacement Therapy for Hot Flashes

Most women expect to have a hot flash sometime in their lives; after all, it's the most frequent and widely known symptom of menopause. But getting a flash while you're still young and menstruating can be surprising, puzzling, and even frightening, particularly if you've always thought—and many women do—that hot flashes never occur until after menopause. Happily, up-to-the-minute treatments can end hot flashes forever.

Connie had her first hot flash at age thirty-nine. It occurred on a rather eventful occasion: the first day of pre-school for her three-year-old daughter, Emma. Just as Emma

Hot Flashes ... At Your Age?

started to cry inconsolably at the thought of being separated from her mommy, Connie felt a strange and uncomfortable sensation. Suddenly, her heart began to race, her breath quickened, and the skin on her face, arms, and chest felt fiery hot, as if she were standing beside a five-hundred-degree oven in a windowless kitchen on a sweltering summer day.

"I was a basket case," Connie recalls. "My daughter was screaming; I was sweating. I felt like I was losing it. I felt so hot that I just wanted to unzip my skin and hurl myself into the nearest snowbank!"

Connie's flash lasted less than two minutes, but when it was over, she felt shaken and distraught. At the time, she chalked the experience up to anxiety and put it out of her mind. It didn't even occur to her that she might have experienced a bona fide hot flash. After all, she still got her period every month and was the mother of a little preschooler, not a menopausal woman well past her childbearing years.

Yet soon after that incident Connie began having a series of night sweats; that is, hot flashes that repeatedly interrupted her sleep. Sometimes she'd awaken so drenched in sweat that she'd have to get up and change her nightgown and bedding. These unwelcome nocturnal interruptions drained her, leaving Connie tired, irritable, and much less patient with her energetic little daughter.

Just as frustrating as the flashes themselves, however, was Connie's inability to convince her doctor to take her problem seriously. Since she was so young and still menstruating regularly, her physician never even considered the possibility of premenopausal hot flashes. Instead, he blamed the problem on stress and prescribed tranquilizers. Connie took the tranquilizers, but her hot flashes continued. When she tried to explain this to her doctor, he listened in polite silence.

Connie had the feeling he felt she was whining, and she definitely didn't want to seem like a whiner.

The story of Leslie has a happier ending. She was only thirty-eight when she began having frequent hot flashes. Though Leslie was still menstruating regularly and was at low risk for premature menopause, the flashes woke her up so often during the night that she was always exhausted. This unending fatigue made it tough for her to keep up with her two- and four-year-old sons and stay focused on her demanding job as a hospital administrator.

"I can't keep this up, Bernie," Leslie told me. "I wake up about three times a night feeling like I'm on fire. A few minutes later, I'm bathed in sweat. This past weekend, the kids were up both nights with nasty ear infections. By Monday morning, I was a wreck. I've been to two other doctors who told me I'm too young to have a hot flash and that I'm just under too much stress. That's nice, but I have two kids to raise and a job I can't afford to quit. Isn't there anything you can do to help? Some pill I can take or something? This isn't a figment of my imagination!"

I reassured Leslie that she wasn't alone: hot flashes are a very real and bothersome problem for many women. Better yet, she didn't have to quit her job or give up her kids to get relief. But before I prescribed anything, I asked her to start keeping a diary in which she noted when the hot flashes occurred and how intense they felt. Charting hot flashes is an effective way to discover any patterns. This, in turn, helps me determine whether the flashes are indeed caused by insufficient or fluctuating estrogen or by some unrelated medical problem. (If you'd like to try this, using the symptoms diary on page 32 will help you get started.)

I also tested Leslie's hormone levels and discovered that her ovaries were putting out low levels of estrogen. To counteract this, I prescribed very small doses of supplemental estrogen that Leslie took only during the first half of her menstrual cycle. But even this tiny dose was enough to boost her estrogen levels to the point where her hot flashes stopped. After months of sleepless nights, Leslie was finally able to get the rest she needed. When I next saw her, she was transformed into a happier and certainly more *rested* working mom.

WHO GETS HOT FLASHES?

If you've never had a hot flash, chances are you will one day—and maybe a good deal sooner than you think! A surprising number of transitional women, including many younger than age forty, experience hot flashes. The results of a study conducted by Columbia University's Fredi Kronenberg, Ph.D., a well-respected researcher in the field of hot flashes, reveal that hot flashes may start earlier and continue longer than is generally recognized by physicians or noted in gynecology textbooks. Between 75 and 80 percent of all women experience hot flashes at some point in their adult lives, according to studies done at Sweden's University of Göteborg in the mid to late 1980s. Significantly, these studies show that at least 60 percent of women experience flashes *before* they reach menopause.

The likelihood of experiencing hot flashes is not the same for everyone. The closer you get to menopause, the greater your chances become. If you check back to figure 2, the chart of transitional symptoms, on page 17, you'll see that women between thirty-five and thirty-nine are only "slightly likely" to have a hot flash. But women forty to forty-four years old are "somewhat likely" and women over forty-five are "highly likely" to have one.

Unfortunately, research into premenopausal hot flashes is relatively scarce, which is why only the most recent gynecology textbooks even mention their existence—and then, only briefly. That's why so many doctors still dismiss transitional women's complaints, telling them the problem is "all in their heads" and claiming that their patients "couldn't possibly" be having hot flashes because they are "way too young" for a symptom that doesn't occur until menopause. The sad fact is that if a thirty-eight-year-old woman tells her gynecologist that she's having night awakenings and heavy sweats, her doctor is much less likely to diagnose the problem as hot flashes than if a fifty-year-old woman offers the same complaints.

Fortunately, however, this situation is beginning to change. Now that doctors are learning more about the special problems of transitional women, such complaints are being taken more seriously. Also, since research now supports what women have long known—that hot flashes are a real and often upsetting physiological phenomenon and not a figment of an overheated imagination—the medical community is paying closer attention.

What Are Hot Flashes?

A hot flash—also called a hot flush, night sweats, or "vasomotor instability," in medical jargon—is a sensation of intense heat, particularly in your upper body. You suddenly begin to feel an overwhelming warmth starting in your chest and moving upward to your shoulders, neck, and face.

While additional symptoms vary from woman to woman, those you might encounter include:

Hot Flashes ... At Your Age?

- *Tingling or numbness in your fingers and toes.*
- *Heart palpitations.*
- *Head pounding or headache.*
- *Chills, either before or after the flash (or both!).*
- *Profuse sweating.*
- *Weakness, faintness, or dizziness.*
- *Anxiety and tension.*

Some women claim they have a premonition of a hot flash—"I could just sense it coming"—just prior to its onset. Others are caught completely off guard. Typically, hot flashes last for about four minutes, but they range in length from thirty seconds to five minutes.

Hot flashes occur more frequently at night, repeatedly awakening a woman from her sleep. This lack of sleep can make you very tired; it can also cause irritability, difficulty concentrating, and a tendency toward forgetfulness. Some women also report feeling annoyed, frustrated, panicky, and, in extreme cases, even suicidal.

Interestingly, some studies suggest a relationship between stress and hot flashes. In a 1990 Canadian study, for instance, a group of women ages thirty-seven to seventy (almost all of whom were already menopausal) were exposed to various psychological stressors—loud noises, frustrating math tasks that had to be completed within very short time periods, films of gory on-the-job accidents suffered by factory workers, and videotapes of people in heated emotional conflicts. The study showed that these women clearly experienced more hot flashes when they were under emotional strain than when they were calm and relaxed.

Where you live may also affect your hot flashes. Women in hot, humid climates tend to report more intense flashes than those who live in cooler, drier locales. Also, women who live in Japan and Indonesia report fewer hot flashes than women who live in Western societies. Scientists aren't sure what to make of these differences and do not as yet know exactly how climate, geography, or culture influences the frequency or intensity of this annoying symptom.

Here's an interesting tidbit: women aren't the only ones who suffer from hot flashes. Men do, too! Specifically, men who experience a sudden drop in their testosterone level—for example, if they have had a testicle removed or if their sexual organs have defective or insufficient internal secretions—can and do have hot flashes.

How Many Hot Flashes Will You Have?

Once again, how often you get a hot flash varies widely. Some women report only a few per year; others suffer several a day. One study of women ages forty-five to fifty-four (only some of whom were menopausal) found that 70 percent experienced hot flashes daily. But since research concerning hot flashes only in transitional women is virtually nonexistent, it's hard to predict just how often you may be troubled by this problem.

If you're experiencing hot flashes and want to get a better fix on their frequency, chart them for a month or so using the symptoms diary on page 32. This will give you a much clearer picture of your individual situation than relying on your memory, and it will help your doctor prescribe the best treatment.

Lack of research also makes it difficult to guess the number of years your hot flashes will continue. The range is enormous. Studies of menopausal women suggest that, if left untreated, hot flashes can continue anywhere from one to sixteen years. I had a patient who refused to treat her hot flashes until she'd been suffering with them for ten years!

There's no specific age at which a woman may have her first hot flash. Similarly, there's no cutoff point at which her flashes will end. Research does suggest, however, that there may be some connection between when your hot flashes start and how long they'll continue. One study seems to suggest that women who begin having hot flashes early on tend to experience them for a greater number of years than women whose hot flashes begin much later. So if your hot flashes begin at a relatively early age, you may be more inclined to seek treatment, knowing that they could last for years.

Typically, untreated hot flashes continue for about two to five years, and many women say their flashes get shorter and less frequent over time. Still and all, frequency, intensity, and symptomatology vary widely, not only from woman to woman but for each individual as well. You may experience your hot flashes differently from day to day, month to month, even year to year.

What Causes Hot Flashes?

Hot flashes are a sign that a woman's estrogen levels have dropped. When estrogen levels fall abruptly, your body's thermostat, located deep within your brain in the hypothalamus, goes haywire. The hypothalamus interprets the drop in estrogen as a drop in body temperature and responds by triggering mechanisms in your sympathetic nervous system (which controls most of your body's reflex actions) to warm you up. Blood rushes to the skin, causing the intense feeling of heat and the skin flushing that characterize the hot flash.

As the blood vessels start to return to their normal size and excrete their excess fluids, the skin begins to sweat and cool you down.

As you're already aware, estrogen production begins to decline in women after about age thirty-five. Although we don't really understand why, some women seem to be more sensitive than others to this gradual reduction in hormone levels, and their bodies react with hot flashes early on in their lives, long before estrogen levels have dropped low enough to stop menstruation—that is, long before menopause.

In other cases, hot flashes have nothing to do with normal hormonal changes; instead, they have a variety of other causes. Consider this checklist of hot flash inducers:

Weight loss.

Since the body's fat stores are an important source of supplemental estrogen, the thinner you are, the more likely you are to suffer hot flashes. This is one of the main reasons why some athletes experience hot flashes: they train so intensively that nearly all of their fat tissue is converted to muscle, depleting their estrogen levels enough to cause their periods to stop and, for some, hot flashes to occur.

If you've dropped more than a few pounds lately, this alone may have brought about your hot flashes. Sometimes simply gaining back some weight, even as little as five pounds or so, can end the problem.

Medications.

Some drugs list hot flashes as one of their side effects. If your flushes started after you began taking one of these medications, this may be the source of your problem. Among the kinds of drugs that can trigger hot flashes are:

ANTI-ESTROGENS. These hormones reduce or eliminate all the estrogen present in your body. As a result, they often cause women to suffer various menopausal symptoms, including hot flashes. The most commonly prescribed anti-estrogens include:

• *Clomiphene.* This popular fertility drug helps some infertile women conceive. About 10 percent of users get hot flashes as a temporary side effect. If my patients are any indication, however, I'd say more like 20 percent of women taking clomiphene temporarily suffer hot flashes.
• *Tamoxifen.* Frequently prescribed for women who have had breast cancer, this drug may prevent the recurrence of tumors that require estrogen to fuel their growth. It's also being tested in current studies to determine if it can help reduce the risk of breast cancer for certain high-risk women. But while tamoxifen's anti-estrogen properties block the effects of estrogen in target tissues, such as the breast, they may cause hot flashes because of the drug's general anti-estrogen behavior throughout the body, including the brain.
• *Danazol.* A synthetic male hormone, danazol is taken primarily for endometriosis, a condition in which cells similar to those in the lining of the uterus are present in other pelvic areas. Decreasing estrogen levels with an anti-estrogen drug causes these endometrial cells to stop functioning and atrophy, which relieves much of the pain women with endometriosis often experience. Danazol is also prescribed for noncancerous breast lumps or breast pain if the underlying cause is thought to be estrogen. Although the lowered estrogen levels this drug brings about can counter-

act estrogen-related problems, danazol can also trigger hot flashes.

(FYI: Because danazol may cause a number of other unpleasant side effects, such as increased hairiness or skin changes, it's only prescribed if and when milder treatments fail.)

GnRH AGONISTS. GnRH (gonadotropin-releasing hormone) agonists are hormones that prevent GnRH from acting and FSH and LH from being released by the pituitary. They, too, can cause hot flashes. GnRH agonists are often prescribed for endometriosis because they prevent endometrial cells from growing outside of the lining of the uterus. They're also given for fibroids, since it is believed that regular reproductive cycles are what keep fibroids active and these drugs disrupt menstrual cycles, causing women to stop having periods. Widely prescribed GnRH agonists include:

- *Lupron.* This synthetic, injectable hormone not only causes a reduction in estrogen, it may also affect the body's thermostat (hypothalmus), prompting hot flashes to occur.
- *Synerol.* This drug acts identically to Lupron, but it is sniffed, not injected.

ANTIDEPRESSIVE TRANQUILIZERS. You should be aware that certain antidepressive tranquilizers, such as Xanax and Tofranil, may cause nonhormonal hot flashes. Here's why. The nerves in the body are not continuous but connected in a series; biochemicals called monamines send messages from one nerve to the next.

Specifically, a monamine called serotonin is released by the nerves in the temporal lobe of the brain (the part of the brain involved when you feel anxious). Xanax and Tofranil reduce the amount of serotonin in the brain, which causes you to feel less anxious. But these drugs don't just act on the brain; they also reduce the amount of serotonin in the hypothalamus. The hypothalamus interprets this drop in serotonin as a drop in body temperature and reacts by activating mechanisms to warm you up, thus causing a hot flash. If you're taking any of these drugs and have started getting hot flashes, check with your doctor; he or she may want you to reduce your dosage or may advise you to stop taking them altogether. This advice also holds true for certain antihypertensive medications, such as clonidine.

Stress.

Hot flashes have also been linked to periods of acute stress. When you are in a stressful situation—you're asked to give an impromptu speech at an important business meeting, or your four-year-old throws a temper tantrum at your mother-in-law's birthday party—your nervous system becomes hyperstimulated, causing adrenaline to shoot into your bloodstream. The sudden increase of adrenaline triggers your hypothalamus to set in motion the mechanisms of a hot flash. Chronic stress—dealing with an ill and aging parent or a demanding and hard-to-please employer day after day—makes you more vulnerable to acute stressors and more susceptible to the hot flashes they can cause.

Surgical causes of hot flashes.

You might also experience hot flashes after undergoing certain surgeries. If you've had your ovaries removed or surgically damaged, you may suddenly get a hot flash. The reason is that the ovaries produce estrogen; when they are removed, estrogen is abruptly withdrawn, causing the chain reaction I explained earlier.

The removal of your pituitary gland can also trigger hot flashes because it reduces your ovaries' ability to function. Remember, the ovaries get their impetus from gonadotropic hormones that are manufactured in and secreted from the pituitary.

Hot flash impersonators.

Occasionally, what you think is a hot flash may not be one at all. If you have an overactive thyroid gland, for example, it can secrete a surplus of thyroxine, which can make your body temperature rise and cause you to have sudden, profuse sweating that resembles a hot flash. But there's a difference. A "real" hot flash lasts only a few moments and affects the upper body only. The sweating brought about by an overactive thyroid lasts much longer—anywhere from five minutes to two hours—and affects your entire body. (For more information on thyroid disorders, see Chapter Nine.)

If you're a diabetic and suffer a sudden dip in blood sugar, you may get heart palpitations and suddenly feel very hot. We're not exactly sure why this occurs, although the most likely reason is that your metabolism is disturbed. These sensations differ from a real hot flash in that rather than passing quickly, they will continue until you get enough sugar into your body to normalize your blood sugar level. (A few swallows of orange juice, for instance, and the "flash" will end.)

Here's one more good way to tell a "real" hot flash from an impersonator: if, in addition to the flashes, you're also experiencing another symptom associated with lowered estrogen levels, such as intense mood swings or increased vaginal dryness, you're probably having the real thing. That said, let me add that if you experience *any* hot flash sensations, you should consult your doctor. Hot flashes may be a warning of another kind of problem, such as certain types of tumors, diabetic insulin reaction, alcohol withdrawal, or an overabundance of thyroid hormone, and may require medical attention.

Simple Treatments for Hot Flashes

In and of themselves, hormonal hot flashes are harmless and will disappear in time. So if your flushes are so infrequent and minor that they really don't bother you much, you don't need to do anything about them.

I suggest, however, that all my transitional patients keep a symptoms diary like the one on page 32. Carefully noting what you did before your hot flash occurred—what foods you ate, which beverages you drank, whether or not you were emotionally upset—may also help you get a fix on what's causing your hot flashes and a head start on how to cure them.

If you're experiencing hot flashes, see if the following simple and safe steps are helpful:

Pay extra attention to what you eat and drink.

(Don't forget to consider medications you may take either occasionally or regularly.) After Samantha, a forty-three-year-old patient of mine, got her first hot flash, I advised her to keep a diary before starting any treatment. She got her second flash a week later, after drinking a full liter bottle of cola, and her third after downing eight cups of black coffee in a single day. When Samantha cut caffeine out of her diet, she successfully eliminated her hot flashes.

Stay cool.

We know that hot flashes tend to be more severe and frequent when the weather is warm. If you heat up inside when it's hot outside—and again, your symptoms diary should help you find out—try turning up the air conditioner and/or lowering the thermostat to keep yourself cooler.

Relax.

Since you may tend to experience more hot flashes when you're under stress, try to stay calm as much as possible. The stress busters mentioned in Chapter Twelve—including deep breathing, muscle relaxation, guided imagery and visualization, meditation, massage (both giving and getting!), yoga, and hypnosis—reduce the hyperstimulation of your nervous system, including your hypothalamus. Thus, these techniques can do wonders to help you cope with acute and chronic stress and, thus, alleviate your hot flashes. If these approaches aren't sufficient, consider therapy and possibly even medication.

Take vitamin E.

Although there's no medical evidence to support vitamin E as a treatment for hot flashes, some of my patients insist it has helped them. If you want to try it, start out with 400 IU (international unit) once daily; if your flushes don't improve in one week, take the same amount twice a day, preferably after you eat, because E is absorbed better after meals. Be sure to consult with your doctor, though; vitamin E should not be taken if you have any history of blood clots or if you're on certain prescription drugs, such as the anticoagulant coumarin, since the vitamin can counteract the effects of some medications.

Exercise.

I once had a patient who walked eight miles a day during her three-week vacation. Although she had flashes before and after her trip, during the holiday she was flash-free. I've heard many such stories touting exercise as an effective hot flash treatment, and as long as you don't overdo it, I'd advise you to give it a whirl. Aerobic exercise, such as walking, hiking, and swimming, seems to be the most effective and, as long as it's done in moderation, can't do any harm. Again, always check with your doctor before beginning any exercise regimen.

HORMONE REPLACEMENT THERAPY FOR HOT FLASHES

You may find that the simple, more natural treatments we've discussed only bring partial relief or, in some cases, no relief at all. Take heart. Many women have found great relief from today's latest medical treatments, particularly hormone replacement therapy.

Birth control pills (BCP).

As I discussed in Chapter Three, birth control pills are a form of hormone replacement therapy. Today's low-dose BCP contains a combination of synthetic hormones that compensate for age-related fluctuations in your hormone levels. With BCP you no longer have to depend on the supply of estrogen and progesterone produced by your own ovaries. Thus, when you take the Pill, you're unlikely to experience any menopausal symptoms—including hot flashes—that your failing ovaries would normally trigger. (However, some women find that when they take BCP, they initially get hot flashes for a short period of time.) In addition, of course, you get excellent protection from unwanted pregnancy.

We've already discussed the benefits of today's Pill: it cuts your risk for endometrial cancer, regulates your menstrual cycle, and helps prevent hormonal cysts of the ovaries. I feel so good about today's BCP that I regularly recommend it to my transitional patients who want to stop their hot flashes cold. Those women who choose to stay on the Pill right through menopause find they *never* experience any of the problems associated with that potentially trying stage of life.

An actress I know came into my office for a routine checkup when she turned forty. "Bernie," she asked when her exam was over, "is there any way to skip menopause altogether?" Although she was chuckling as she asked, I sensed she was serious. After all, she was in a highly image-conscious business and I knew she must have been very concerned about looking older. In addition, the thought of having a hot flash onstage before hundreds of people was horrifying to her!

Since she was in excellent health and didn't want any more kids—she was already the mother of two school-aged youngsters—I told her that taking birth control pills could virtually eliminate premenopausal problems forever. That's when she started on BCP.

Today she is forty-nine and still taking the Pill; her twice-a-year checkups reveal her to be a young, vital woman who is still in top condition. To date, she's never suffered a hot flash, menstrual problems, mood swings, or any of the other symptoms associated with menopause. And she publicly proclaims herself to be in her early forties! (I'll never tell.)

Eventually, I'll probably recommend a regimen of hormone replacement therapy in which estrogen dosages are even lower than those of the Pill. I will do this when she goes into menopause, although this is not as easy as it sounds because the BCP will allow her to make such a smooth transition into menopause she will not have any of the usual telltale symptoms. Therefore, I'll take my cues from either her family history (and change her treatment when she reaches the age at which her mother went into menopause) or from demographics (and switch her to lower estrogen dosages at about age fifty, the age at which most women become menopausal). I'm confident that whenever this happens, she'll never suffer any symptoms of menopause—other than the eventual loss of her period.

Will the BCP approach work for you? That depends on your health, your family medical history, and your own attitude about taking hormones for so many years. But I believe that if you're carefully screened by a qualified physician before you begin—and if you conscientiously have regular checkups—this treatment can be both safe and highly effective.

Estrogen therapy.

Since hot flashes are triggered by lowered estrogen levels, it makes sense that replacing your estrogen would be an excellent form of treatment. Many women mistakenly believe that the closer they are to menopause, the more estrogen they need. In fact, only small quantities of estrogen are required—actually one tenth the amount found in birth control pills—to prevent hot flashes. These minimal amounts of estrogen are the basis of estrogen supplement therapy (EST).

So if you're between thirty-five and forty-four, taking a tiny dose of supplemental estrogen, similar to the amount you can take to regulate your menstrual cycles, can be very effective. Since hot flashes will usually occur during and immediately after your period, the time in your cycle when estrogen is relatively low, you need to take this minimal dose from the third to the tenth day of your cycle.

If you're over forty-five, still menstruating, and don't want to take the Pill, you could consider more traditional estrogen replacement therapy (ERT). Women younger than forty-five usually don't need full-fledged ERT because their bodies are still producing at least a helpful amount of estrogen. With ERT, you take estrogen from the first to the twenty-fifth day of your cycle, adding progesterone during the last ten days to protect your uterus. (If you no longer have a uterus, you won't need the progesterone.)

ERT is available in a variety of forms—pills, estrogen-releasing skin patches, vaginal creams, or injections—one of which will be right for you. Even so, deciding whether or not to start ERT is not easy. You'll first need to weigh a few health factors.

If there's nothing in your medical history to prevent your taking estrogen, it can work wonders. As I mentioned in Chapter Three, however, you should avoid estrogen if you're pregnant, since it can increase the chance of birth defects; if you have any heart or circulation problems, including abnormal blood clotting and stroke; if you have a history of liver tumors or cancer; or if you smoke. If you do start estrogen therapy, you must have annual medical check-ups, and you should ask your doctor to reevaluate your need for estrogen every six months. Too, you should let your physician know right away if you notice anything unusual, such as abnormal vaginal bleeding or chest pain.

Debbie is an EST success story. At thirty-nine, she was extremely upset by the hot flashes she'd been experiencing for the past four months. "Bernie, I can't believe this is happening to me. I'm only thirty-nine! Could I be going into menopause already? What does this mean?"

According to the symptoms diary she'd kept, Debbie's flashes were quite frequent, occurring nearly every day for a couple of weeks after each period. As Debbie and I talked more, it became clear to me that she was not heading into early menopause; instead, her body was just taking a much longer time to increase its estrogen levels enough to bring about ovulation. That's what was causing her hot flashes.

As she was in excellent health otherwise, but very distressed over the flashes, I recommended estrogen therapy, and she jumped at the chance to get some relief. I prescribed small doses of estrogen daily from day three to day ten of her cycle, and within a month her flashes stopped. Since taking estrogen might cause her to ovulate, she used a diaphragm and contraceptive jelly to avoid a surprise pregnancy. After six months of flash-free living, Debbie decided to become pregnant. At that point, we stopped the estrogen; less than a year later, she had a healthy baby boy whom she nursed for seven months before going back to work full-time. At this point, her own normal cycles have resumed, and thus far she's remained free from flashes. Should they return, however, we will discuss treatment.

Progesterone therapy.

Although some women complain about progesterone's possible side effects—breast tenderness, bloating, irritability, occasional nausea, insomnia, or even a slight increase in light facial or body hair—progesterone can be an effective remedy for hot flashes because it enhances estrogen action. Your doctor may prescribe either MPA, a popular oral progestin, which you would take on day thirteen of your cycle and continue for ten to thirteen days, or a low-progestin birth control pill that you would take for the entire month.

Remember, progesterone therapy varies with the problem being treated. As I discussed in Chapter Three, to fix menstrual problems, progesterone is given in a manner that will allow it to counteract the effect of high estrogen levels and to protect the endometrial lining from overgrowth. To alleviate hot flashes, progesterone is given in such a way as to enhance estrogen.

Not everyone is a good candidate for progesterone therapy, however. Women with any vascular problems such as blood clots, or those who have liver problems, cancers of the breast or genital organs, unexplained vaginal bleeding, or, of course, women who are pregnant, should avoid progestins. After you begin treatment, be sure to tell your doctor immediately if you experience any chest or leg pain, loss of vision, migraine headaches, or if you become pregnant. But if progesterone is right for you, it can offer wonderful relief.

Anti–hot flash drugs.

I've found hormonal treatments are generally best for ending hot flashes. But if they don't work for you—or if, for whatever reason, you *can't* or *won't* try them—you still have a few other options. Depending on your current health and personal medical history, you may get relief from certain anti–hot flash drugs. These include the following:

- *Clonidine.* Usually prescribed for high blood pressure, clonidine, which you can take either in pill form or through a patch, works by controlling nerve impulses along certain nerve pathways of your sympathetic nervous system. As a result, it relaxes the blood vessels so that your blood can pass through more easily.

Since your blood vessels dilate and constrict irregularly during a hot flash, it's not surprising that clonidine helps with this annoying symptom. But because this drug was really not developed for hot flashes—it relieves them only as a side benefit—and because clonidine may cause drowsiness, dizziness, or dry mouth, I don't recommend it for hot flashes unless you need it to control your blood pressure as well.

• *Ergotamine drugs* (such as Cafergot). This class of drugs is usually very effective in treating hot flashes. But they have a major downside: because they act on your sympathetic nervous system, which controls your involuntary muscles, ergotamine drugs can cause uterine contractions and difficulty breathing, as well as hypertension, problems with coronary arteries, hyperthyroidism, and kidney damage. Sometimes the pain and danger of the side effects outweigh the discomfort of the flash itself.

• *Bellergal-S*. Although it contains ergotamine, Bellergal-S is a combination of three different drugs: phenobarbital, ergotamine, and alkaloids of belladonna. In combination, these drugs counteract some of the negative effects of ergotamine, making Bellergal-S a pretty effective treatment for hot flashes. I generally prescribe it for patients with breast and ovarian cancers who cannot take estrogen.

Bonnie, age forty-two, is a case in point. She'd been diagnosed with breast cancer. Luckily, it was a localized carcinoma of the right breast that was removed with a lumpectomy; there was no evidence that the cancer had spread. Since Bonnie's tumor was estrogen-dependent, she went on tamoxifen, an anti-estrogen medication, immediately after surgery. (For more on estrogen and cancer, see Chapter Ten).

In terms of the cancer, Bonnie's prognosis was quite good.

However, since anti-estrogen drugs such as tamoxifen reduce or even eliminate all estrogen present in the body, she became menopausal and started having intense and frequent hot flashes. Obviously, Bonnie could not begin hormone therapy, so I prescribed daily doses of Bellergal-S, which reduced the number of flashes almost immediately. It has taken several weeks, however, for the remaining flashes to become less intense. Bonnie will keep taking Bellergal-S until her flashes disappear; after about a year, we may try reducing the dose level.

While Bonnie hasn't suffered any side effects whatsoever, the drug has its downside. Bellergal-S doesn't interact well with many other drugs, so if you're taking other medications simultaneously, you may have some problems. It's important to make sure you give your doctor a complete list of any other medications you may already be taking before you start on Bellergal-S. One more negative: this drug can be habit-forming, another reason I only prescribe it when other treatments either fail or aren't appropriate.

- *Tranquilizers.* I include tranquilizers as a form of treatment for hot flashes only because some doctors still prescribe them for this purpose. But I believe it's the wrong way to go. Tranquilizers have such a global effect on your nervous system that I find their use difficult to justify in women who have only one symptom they wish to alleviate. It's like taking a multiaction cold remedy—one that works to relieve fever, coughing, congestion, and a runny nose—when all you have is a bad cough.

A Closing Word

Hot flashes. A figment of your imagination? A problem you'll just have to learn to live with? Hardly. Instead, they're a real and highly treatable symptom of the changes

Hot Flashes . . . At Your Age?

that affect many transitional women. If you're bothered by persistent hot flashes but don't want to be, insist that your doctor take your complaint seriously and work with you to bring about the relief you deserve.

5

Birth Control After Thirty-Five

- The Downside of Pregnancy and Childrearing Later in Life
- Barrier Methods of Birth Control
- Birth Control Pills
- Injections
- Implants
- The Intrauterine Device (IUD)
- Natural Methods
- Surgical Approaches
- Avoiding a "Surprise" Pregnancy

Deciding whether or not to have a baby can be one tough choice, particularly for a woman in her transitional years. While your biological clock certainly hasn't wound down completely—in fact, Chapter Six tells you how to keep it ticking through your mid-forties—time is no longer on your side. You realize, and accurately so, that you won't stay fertile forever and that if you want to get pregnant you need to make a decision relatively soon.

As a reproductive endocrinologist, I've chosen to devote much of my life's work to helping women have happy, healthy babies for as long as they possibly can. But I also see many patients who are very clear about *not* wanting to get pregnant. If you are sexually active but would like to avoid pregnancy—for now or forever—this chapter is for you.

The Downside of Pregnancy and Childrearing Later in Life

Below age thirty-five, giving birth offers some important health benefits. Since the early seventies, we have known that having a baby when you're in your twenties cuts your risk for breast cancer. If you breast-feed your baby, your chances of developing the disease drop even further. What's more, we find that young women who have experienced pregnancy and childbirth have healthier hearts after delivery than they did before they got pregnant—for the very same reason that regular aerobic workouts can improve your cardiovascular health.

Pregnancy and delivery are also easier on a younger woman. When you're in your twenties, your muscles are young, strong, and quite able to withstand the stress of pregnancy and childbirth. A younger body is also more able to tolerate the many other physiological shifts of childbearing, including changes in blood sugar levels, blood pressure, and the added strain on the heart and lungs.

Once you reach your late thirties and your forties, however, you face more medical drawbacks. Even if you're in pretty good shape, your bones, muscles, heart, and lungs are older and thus less able to tolerate the extra wear and tear. If you're over thirty-five, you're also more likely to experience much more dramatic changes in blood sugar and blood pressure than you would have a few years earlier.

You also may have less overall energy, particularly if you haven't followed the guidelines offered in my ten-point health plan (see page 30). Reduced stamina makes it harder to go through pregnancy as well as to meet the needs of a demanding infant and, eventually, an energetic toddler.

Transitional women also run a greater risk of miscarriage and fetal loss. A thirty-five-year-old woman is more likely to suffer a miscarriage than a younger woman, and a woman of forty is likelier still. What's more, certain medical conditions that are more common in women over thirty-five—such as diabetes—can be aggravated by pregnancy.

After age forty, the risk for toxemia of pregnancy, or preeclampsia, a condition marked by hypertension, edema (swelling, usually of the feet, ankles, and hands), and headaches, increases dramatically. A review of studies, published in the *Obstetrical and Gynecologic Survey* of 1988, reveals that while the risk for toxemia is only 4 percent in pregnant women between the ages of thirty-five and thirty-nine, that number jumps to 41 percent after age forty. If not treated properly—usually with bed rest and plenty of fluids—preeclampsia can lead to seizures in the mother or even coma, induction of labor, or cesarean section.

Finally, if you need to rely on fertility drugs to help you conceive, you stand a higher chance of having a multiple birth, which can be risky for you and your babies. Multiple births are more likely to trigger hypertension, preeclampsia, and premature delivery.

Then there's the infant's health to consider. Most transitional women give birth to perfectly healthy babies, but after age thirty-five the risk for certain congenital problems increases. For example, while the chance of having a baby born with Down's syndrome is less than 5 percent at age thirty-five, that number shoots to 15 percent by the time you reach forty. Researchers at the University of Washington in Seattle studied thousands of women over thirty-five who gave birth to their first babies between 1984 and 1988 and found that their babies had a higher risk for low birth weight and prematurity than babies born to younger mothers—*and* that this risk increased progressively with the mother's age. Today many medical problems can be detected and managed effectively during pregnancy, but overall, the baby of a transitional woman is at higher risk.

Aside from the physical disadvantages we've already discussed, becoming a mom in your transitional years has some psychological drawbacks also. If you wind up traveling the infertility route—and the older you are, the greater the likelihood that you'll need some help getting pregnant—you may find yourself on an emotional roller coaster. While each new treatment can make your hopes soar, each failure—such as artificial inseminations that don't take, surgery that doesn't help, repeated miscarriage, or high-tech procedures that just don't work for you—can send your spirits crashing again. These ups and downs, hopes and disappointments, take an enormous toll, causing tension between you and your mate and in all likelihood making you feel unwomanly, depressed, and inadequate.

Even if your time and effort pay off and you're able to have the baby you so desperately wanted, you may find that motherhood has some unpleasant psychological surprises. As thirty-nine-year-old Elaine told me, "I wanted a baby so badly I could taste it. But somehow, I just never really thought about the day-to-dayness of caring for her. I got so caught up in the idea of having a beautiful little infant, all soft and sweet and cuddly, I never really stopped to think about the crying, lack of sleep, midnight feedings, and diaper changes.

"Even more, I've suddenly discovered that I'm not my own person anymore; I always have this other totally dependent little being to think about. Don't get me wrong. I love my baby and I can't imagine my life without her. But I have to admit that suddenly being this tied down has been a bit of a shock—and an unpleasant one at that."

The restriction of freedom that's part and parcel of being a mom can hit hard if you're in your transitional years. When you were childless—or "child-free," as many women without kids prefer to be called—you could pretty much come and go as you pleased. With a child, however, you have the constant care of another to consider. After twenty years or so of being their own bosses, some women don't want to give up their independence.

Having a baby may also prevent you from devoting as much time and attention to your career as you have been. I'm not saying that motherhood means giving up your work. It's just that you may not be able to work with the same devotion, intensity, or relish you had in the past. A brand-new baby in the house may mean putting your career on hold for a while, or at least cutting back for a few years. This is not an easy pill for some women to swallow, especially those who have already invested the past decade or two building a career that in large part defines who they are.

Even if you can afford to hire help, balancing the conflicting demands of career and family can be emotionally and physically exhausting. Working mothers often live in a constant state of guilt: when they're at home, they feel guilty that they're not working; when they're at the office, they agonize over what they are missing at home. This is an ongoing dilemma for working mothers, but it is most acute when they feel their child's babyhood is speeding by.

If you're married or have lived with the same partner for a number of years without children, adding a child to your love nest can ruffle more than a few feathers. Male partners often feel neglected by mates who seem to devote all their time and attention to this newcomer—and they don't like it.

But men don't have the corner on resentment. New moms often feel their mates aren't pulling their weight, and research backs them up. Surveys of American couples have shown that even when both partners work, the woman still gets stuck with the lion's share of baby-related and household chores.

Women in their transitional years also worry about something most younger women don't: the future. If you have your children when you're in your twenties, they'll be grown by the time you reach your forties. You'll have your childrearing chores behind you when you still have half of your life ahead of you, which gives you an average of thirty or even forty years to turn your attention to other accomplishments.

Having a child in your mid or late transitional years means you'll be actively parenting when you're a senior citizen—which may put the kibosh on rewards such as early retirement. It's hard to consider a life under the palm trees of Florida or among the red rock vistas of Arizona when you have at least four years of college tuition to think about. True, if you keep yourself healthy and active, you can live well into your seventies, eighties—even your nineties—and still enjoy a long and vital retirement. But unquestionably, having a child when you're in your transitional years does postpone or at least change the nature of your "golden years."

Whether you feel you already have enough children or you choose to remain child-free, birth control after age thirty-five brings with it some special considerations. If you select the right option for you from the choices that follow, you should be able to avoid being put in the position of dealing with a surprise pregnancy in your transitional years.

Barrier Methods of Birth Control

"Barrier" contraceptives are those that prevent the sperm and egg from meeting by covering the cervix or, in the case of condoms, by preventing the sperm from ever reaching the cervix. All barrier methods offer very good protection from pregnancy, usually with no accompanying problems. The biggest drawback is that you have to remember to put the barrier contraceptive in (or on, in the case of condoms) *before* you have intercourse—something that might prevent you from being as spontaneous as you'd like. But the effectiveness and lack of significant side effects of these contraceptives makes them worth considering.

The diaphragm.

This contraceptive device is made of latex rubber with a contouring spring. Since diaphragms come in various sizes, from sixty to ninety millimeters, your doctor must fit you for one; make sure that once it is inserted, you feel no pressure or pain. If you do, it is not the correct size for you. I usually prescribe All-Flex by Ortho, or Koro-Flex by Schmid.

A diaphragm should be kept in for six hours after intercourse, and can be put in up to six hours prior to intercourse. It should always be used with a contraceptive jelly or cream; if intercourse takes place six hours or more after the diaphragm has been inserted, you will need to reapply the spermicidal jelly or cream to make sure you're still protected.

The contraceptive sponge.

This device is a soft polyurethane foam sponge that contains a spermicide for twenty-four-hour protection from unwanted pregnancy. One size fits all, so you can buy it over the counter without a doctor's prescription. It's also disposable; you use it once, then toss it out. The one I recommend is the Today brand (although it may be difficult to find).

There are very few side effects associated with the contraceptive sponge, although some people have a sensitivity to the spermicide. You do have to be careful not to leave it in too long, however, because if you do you may become vulnerable to toxic shock syndrome (TSS). Symptoms include fever, vomiting, diarrhea, muscular pain, dizziness, and a sunburnlike rash.

Contraceptive foam and inserts.

Some spermicides are made to be used alone. Inserts such as Spermicid or contraceptive foam used alone act as a barrier to sperm during sexual intercourse. Since these products aren't as effective in preventing pregnancy as other barrier methods, and don't provide any protection against STDs, I don't recommend them.

The cervical cap.

If you desire, your doctor can fit you with a cervical cap. When inserted properly, this latex rubber device fits so snugly over the cervix that no spermicide is necessary. But because the fit is so tight, it's tricky to insert correctly—and if it's not precisely in place, it can dislodge and leave you unprotected. For this reason, I recommend that women who choose the cervical cap use it with contraceptive foam or cream, at least until they become skilled at putting it in correctly.

Condoms.

The other key barrier method—and the only contraceptive device that can be used by the male partner—is the condom, a sheath made of latex, sheepskin, or lamb's gut that fits over a man's penis. The condom has a similar downside to other barrier methods—it's hard to be spontaneous—or, I might add, graceful—when you're putting one on. But it also has a considerable upside: effective protection not only against pregnancy but also against STDs and AIDS.

I recommend latex condoms because they provide the best and most reliable protection against pregnancy *and* disease, since the organisms that cause STDs and AIDS cannot penetrate latex but can get through lamb gut or sheepskin. The thin (as opposed to thick) variety will allow the man to feel more sensation during intercourse, and lubricated versions may be more comfortable for transitional women whose vaginal secretions are declining, but overall, the style you get—whether straight or tapered, smooth or ribbed, colored or clear, lubricated or nonlubricated—is a matter of individual preference.

Today, there's also a female condom available that fits into the vagina and protects the cervix. While the jury's still out on how popular it will become, early reports suggest there seem to be some problems with fit, slippage, and the disconcerting noise it sometimes makes during intercourse.

Birth Control Pills

You may have assumed that you are too old to take birth control pills, but thanks to today's new formulations, which contain far lower and safer hormone dosages, you may be able to take the Pill throughout your transitional years, all the way until menopause. Birth control pills not only offer nearly 100 percent protection from unwanted pregnancy, but also, as I've discussed in earlier chapters, help alleviate many premenopausal complaints. They help to regulate your periods—an important benefit for those of you bothered by menstrual irregularity. Equally important is the fact that the extra estrogen you get with the Pill can prevent many of the premenopausal symptoms you may otherwise suffer during your transitional years, including intensified PMS, dry vagina, and mood swings. (To help decide if the Pill is safe for you, see my discussion of the Pill in Chapter Three.)

Injections

A long-acting progestin called Depo-Provera has recently been introduced into the U.S. market. Injected into the gluteal muscle of the backside every three months, the progestin is released continuously over that time period. It works by reducing the ability of estrogen to cycle. Depo-Provera is a convenient method of birth control, since you need an injection only four times a year.

But the product has some drawbacks. It does not protect you against sexually transmitted diseases and often causes irregular or unpredictable bleeding as well as weight gain.

Use of this contraceptive has also been associated with increased risk for osteoporosis. Since many transitional women are already suffering from menstrual irregularity and a weakening of bone strength, I do not recommend it for women over age thirty-five. However, if you do not like or for some reason cannot use any other form of birth control, Depo-Provera could be considered.

Implants

Another birth control option is levonorgestrel implants. The type I prescribe is Norplant. Introduced in this country in 1991, Norplant is a long-acting hormonal contraceptive that's implanted under the skin of your upper arm during a quick office procedure. Only a local anesthetic is needed.

Once implanted, Norplant slowly releases progesterone into your system and in doing so prevents ovulation. Once in place, the implant can protect you from pregnancy for up to five years. It's also completely reversible; the implant can be readily removed if you no longer want protection from unwanted pregnancy.

As for side effects, some women experience some menstrual irregularity, but this usually diminishes within a year. Because Norplant delivers progesterone, it sometimes causes other side effects similar to those some women experience with progesterone therapy, including breast tenderness, irritability, nausea, and bloating. Norplant differs from progesterone therapy, however, in that it offers a constant outflow of progesterone so that you maintain a persistent level of the hormone in your bloodstream at all times. (Oral progestins used in progesterone therapy provide short bursts of the hormone only on certain days of your cycle.) But this persistence can lead to headaches and dizziness in some women. Also, removal does require additional minor surgery. Norplant isn't recommended for women who have acute liver disease, unexplained vaginal bleeding, breast cancer, or a history of blood clots in the legs, lungs, or eyes.

THE INTRAUTERINE DEVICE (IUD)

Most IUDs are small, flexible devices, usually made of plastic and copper, and may have progesterone embedded in them. The IUD is inserted into the uterus in a process similar to an endometrial biopsy. During a quick and relatively painless office procedure, a tube that contains the collapsed IUD is introduced into the uterus through the cervix. The IUD is then pushed out of the tube and unfolds in the uterus, and the tube is withdrawn. The nylon string(s) that are attached to the IUD protrude through the cervical opening, allowing you to regularly check to make sure that the IUD is still in place. The string(s) also provide your doctor with a simple means for removing the device when necessary.

Although the IUD is an effective contraceptive device, ever since the Dalkon Shield disaster, in which many women suffered permanent intrauterine damage, women have been wary of it. It's important to realize, though, that today's models are quite safe and effective. Depending on the type of IUD you choose, the same device can work for three to seven years. The one I like best is ParaGard, made by GynoPharma, a T-shaped device made of plastic wrapped with copper wire that is comfortable for the patient and easy for the doctor to insert.

Using an IUD does require some vigilance, however. If you use one, you should see your gynecologist every six months—immediately if you notice any abdominal bloating or unusual vaginal discharge. The reason is that users may be more prone to infection.

Here's why: if you don't have an IUD and you get an infection, that infection usually stays localized and can be easily treated. With an IUD, a small, local infection can quickly spread through the cervix to the uterus and into your fallopian tubes, creating a much more difficult and potentially dangerous problem called pelvic inflammatory disease (PID). If left untreated, PID can cause an infection that would require hospitalization to treat, damage your pelvic organs, and possibly leave you permanently sterile.

Although we're not exactly sure why IUD users are at higher risk for PID, one theory is that an IUD that chronically irritates the uterus could leave you more vulnerable to fresh STD infection. Another possibility is that bacteria can be carried on the device and spread from the vagina to the uterus and tubes. Whatever the cause, if not caught in its earliest stages, PID can be dangerous, so be sure to have your doctor check your IUD every six months—sooner, if you feel any pelvic or abdominal discomfort.

You should also be aware of the fact that some women's bodies don't tolerate the IUD and expel it—occasionally without the woman's even realizing it's gone—within the first three months after insertion. Even more rarely, the IUD may perforate the uterus and could even maneuver its way into the abdomen. To make sure that the IUD is in and in place, be sure to check the string(s) periodically; if you can't find them, see your doctor immediately.

Another problem is that women who have had an IUD and then try to become pregnant are at greater risk for ectopic pregnancy, possibly because of problems arising from previous infections, some of which they may not ever have known about. For this reason, I do not recommend the IUD for women who plan on having children. You should also not use an IUD if you have PID, known or suspected uterine or cervical cancer, an infection, abnormal Pap smear results, or genital bleeding for which you don't know the cause.

Natural Methods

Basal body temperature.

Some women prefer to use natural methods of birth control, which work by determining the best times *not* to have intercourse because it is at these times that you are most likely to become pregnant. One such method relies on your basal body temperature. You simply take your temperature for five minutes as soon as you get up each morning and record your reading on a chart like the one offered on page 134. Start a new chart the first day of your period.

After several days, you should notice your temperature drop and then abruptly rise the next morning by one half to one degree; this means that you may be ovulating and should not have intercourse at this time.

If you take your temperature every single day, after about two to three months you should begin to see a pattern and to have a good idea about when you ovulate. Once you do, you should abstain from having intercourse from forty-eight hours before ovulation to forty-eight hours after.

A few words of caution. If you ovulate irregularly, and thus cannot predict your ovulation accurately each month, then this is not a good birth control option for you. Also understand that sperm can stay alive inside you for as long as seven days, so even if you ovulate at the exact same time each month and are diligent about abstaining during your most fertile times, this is not a 100 percent foolproof method of birth control.

Cervical mucus test.

Up until a few years ago, women could purchase a kit that would allow them to test their cervical mucus in order to figure out when they were least likely to get pregnant. Here's how it worked: after taking their basal body temperature for a couple of months to get a sense of when they would ovulate, they would take a sample of their cervical mucus each day for a few days before and during ovulation. As they came closer to ovulating, the mucus would become clearer and thinner, or change color on a testing paper.

For various reasons, the test has fallen out of favor and, to my knowledge, is no longer commercially (or at least easily) available. If you choose, however, your doctor can do a cervical mucus test for you.

SURGICAL APPROACHES

Surgery is an extremely effective approach to birth control. But although operations can sometimes be "reversed," you or your partner should not entertain the idea of surgery unless you are *certain* you don't want any (or any more) children.

Surgery for you: tubal ligation.

When Tamara, age forty, walked into my office complaining of mood swings and hot flashes, she hardly seemed like an obvious candidate for early menopause. She had never smoked, was in excellent overall health, and, as an avid tennis player, got plenty of regular exercise. Moreover, her mother and maternal grandmother had gone through menopause relatively late in life, when they were in their mid-fifties.

But Tamara's medical history revealed a significant clue to her problem: three years earlier, she'd had a tubal ligation, a form of permanent sterilization in which the surgeon blocks the fallopian tubes so that the egg and sperm can't meet.

Although tubal ligation (usually called "having your tubes tied") is by far the most popular method of birth control in women over thirty-five—nearly 600,000 American women undergo this surgery every year—I have some strong reservations about it. The reason is that in some women, tubal ligation may reduce estrogen and progesterone production, triggering menstrual problems and speeding up the onset of premenopausal symptoms.

The procedure itself is not complicated. The surgeon opens the pelvic cavity, usually through a tiny incision in the abdomen, and operates on the two fallopian tubes. The doctor generally uses one of two approaches. The first is *laparoscopy*, in which a very small incision is made in the navel through which a device called a laparoscope is inserted. The doctor inserts tiny, specially designed operating instruments through the laparoscope that he or she uses to operate on the tube. The other approach is a *mini-laparotomy*, in which the surgeon makes a one- or two-inch incision just below the pubic hairline and operates directly in the abdomen. In both cases, the doctor closes off the fallopian tubes, which normally act as conduits to carry the egg to the sperm. The tubes are closed off either by cutting and ligation (tying), using plastic clips, or by electrocauterization (burning). Thereafter, when the ovary releases an egg each month, it simply floats away into the abdominal cavity and disintegrates.

We now know that the ovaries can be indirectly affected by tubal ligation. Blood vessels to the ovaries lie very close to the fallopian tubes. If these are inadvertently cut or damaged during surgery, the blood supply to the ovaries may be reduced. Without normal delivery of oxygen and nutrients to nourish the ovaries, they may begin to age prematurely, accelerating the onset of menopause.

There's a lot of controversy over just how often this complication, known as *post–tubal ligation syndrome*, occurs. But I don't really care. Since other contraceptive approaches are available that are noninvasive and don't have the potential of harming your ovaries, I seldom endorse tubal ligation as the best alternative.

I realize, however, that when all goes well, tubal ligation offers a tremendous contraceptive freedom. What's more, a recent study by researchers at Brigham and Women's Hospital in Boston tracked thousands of premenopausal women for over a decade and showed that, all other risk factors being equal, those who had tubal sterilizations were one third as likely as other women to develop ovarian cancer. So I wouldn't go so far as to steer everyone away from the procedure. But if you're thinking about getting your tubes tied, you should consider *all* the pros and cons. And be sure to talk to your surgeon about possible complications that can occur during or after surgery, such as infection, allergic reactions to the anesthesia, or adhesions (scarred tissue). If you opt for tubal sterilization, I believe that a mini-laparotomy using plastic clips is the safest procedure. I don't like electrocauterization, because I feel it is more likely to damage surrounding tissues.

Surgery for him: vasectomy.

Every year, nearly twice as many women as men undergo permanent sterilization. Yet from a medical point of view, vasectomy is a far safer procedure because it doesn't involve opening the abdominal cavity and it doesn't pose any risk to hormone production.

FIGURE 3. *Side View of Male Reproductive Anatomy*

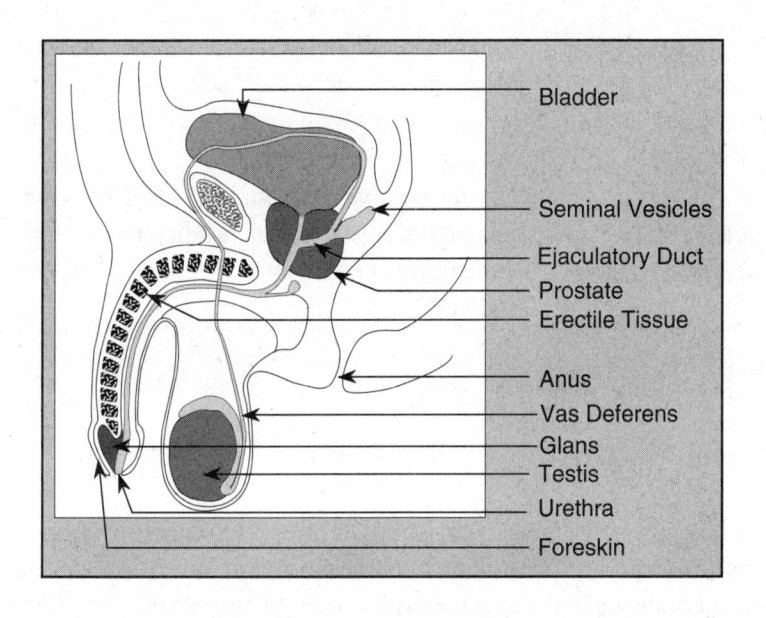

Here's how the procedure works. The *vas deferens*, a tube that begins near the testes, carries the sperm to the ejaculatory ducts (see figure 3). In a vasectomy, a small portion of the vas deferens in the scrotal area is removed so that no sperm reaches the ducts and, therefore, the ejaculate carries no sperm. A vasectomy is done in a doctor's office under local anesthetic.

While vasectomy has very few medical complications, studies done in the United States, including a 1992 study cited in the *Journal of the American Medical Association*, show that men who have had a vasectomy appear to be at a *slightly* increased risk—less than 2 percent—for prostate cancer. However, a 1993 article published in the *Bulletin of the World Health Organization* disputes these findings, asserting that while there is an increased incidence of prostate cancer in the United States overall, there is not enough evidence to link vasectomy with higher risk for the disease.

A much less controversial drawback centers on the fact that reversing the procedure is not always successful or even recommended. Therefore, men who may want children in the future should not have a vasectomy.

One more point: many men won't consider vasectomy because they fear it will interfere with their ability to have an erection. Medically speaking, vasectomy should have no effect on erections whatsoever.

Avoiding a "Surprise" Pregnancy

These days we hear a great deal about the plight of women who desperately want to become pregnant but cannot seem to conceive. In fact, infertility has become such a widespread problem among women in their transitional years that I've devoted Chapter Six entirely to discussing ways to enhance and stretch your fertility.

What gets a lot less publicity, however, are the unplanned pregnancies that occur during the transitional years. I'm sure many of these "surprises" happen because the sexual partner who is taking the responsibility for birth control forgoes that duty during certain sexual encounters. It is also true that no birth control method offers 100 percent protection.

But what concerns me even more is that some transitional women may be laboring under the misconception that after age thirty-five they cannot become pregnant or that the chances are so slim that they don't warrant the inconvenience of birth control. Let me set the record straight: as long as you're still menstruating, you can become pregnant, particularly if you're menstruating regularly. There are signs that indicate that you may become pregnant, including experiencing such premenstrual symptoms as breast tenderness, mild bloating, or mood changes; feeling some minor pain near one or both of your ovaries around mid-cycle; or having an increased amount of vaginal lubrication in the middle of your cycle.

While the chances of becoming pregnant become slimmer for women in their transitional years, slimmer doesn't mean nonexistent. So if you don't want any more kids, or choose to remain child-free, make sure you use the birth control method of your choice every time you have sexual intercourse.

6

How to Enhance—and Stretch—Your Fertility

- How Much Time Do You Have Left?
- Why It's Hard to Get Pregnant Later in Life
- How to Protect Your Fertility
- The Prepregnancy Checkup
- Conceiving the Natural Way
- Checking—and Correcting—Your Anatomy
- How to Fix an Anatomical Problem
- Checking—and Correcting—Your Cycles
- Male Infertility
- How to Correct Male Infertility
- High-Tech Solutions to Infertility Problems
- When You Can't Give Birth to Your Own Baby

Having a baby can be incredibly rewarding and fulfilling. Watching your child grow and develop from infancy and toddlerhood through the school ages, adolescence, and finally young adulthood can be gratifying beyond measure. As the father of three now grown children, I can attest to that personally. Parenthood can open sides of yourself (and your partner) that you may never have known existed, such as a deep capacity for love, devotion, and selflessness.

Transitional women do have concerns that younger mothers don't, as we discussed in Chapter Five. However, many transitional women tell me that their age is an advantage. They believe their years of experience have given them more emotional maturity and patience—two traits essential to effective parenting. As Darleen, a thirty-eight-year-old patient of mine, put it, "I don't think I would have been as good a mom if I'd had my daughter earlier. And I certainly know I wouldn't have enjoyed it as much. Before, I was too caught up in myself; now, my top priority is Ashley."

As a reproductive endocrinologist—or "fertility specialist," as I'm often called—I know that you can extend your fertile years longer than we ever thought possible. In my experience, a healthy transitional woman can continue to conceive and, with proper prenatal care, safely bear a child well into her mid-forties. I had one patient who had a strong, healthy baby—her thirteenth—at age forty-nine!

How Much Time Do You Have Left?

When thirty-nine-year-old Randi came to see me, she was clearly agitated. A computer expert who had managed to break through the academic glass ceiling, she'd recently been named dean of a large university. Her husband, forty-seven-year-old Ron, is a successful real estate broker. Both Randi and Ron enjoy their work and their active social life. Yet they'd decided there was one thing missing from their lives: a baby.

In her always direct style, Randi asked me, "How much

time do I have left to get pregnant? You see, I'd really like to wait a couple of years, until I get more experience and tenure with this job. But if I do that, will I be throwing away my chances of having a healthy baby? Or is there some way to stretch my fertility so I can get pregnant after forty?"

I really felt for Randi; I could hear the urgency in her voice. As I painstakingly tried to answer her questions, I couldn't help but think how many times I'd heard them before. For the past two decades or so, ever since today's baby boomers began to face the fact that they would *not* stay young forever and that there really *were* limits to their childbearing years, I have been bombarded with anxious queries from literally hundreds of transitional women. No matter how they broach the subject or express their concerns, the underlying questions are always the same: "How much time have I got, Bernie? How much longer do I have to conceive and bear a child safely?"

No one can predict how long you'll remain fertile—not yet anyway. Scientists are working to develop tests that may help women figure out how many fertile years they have left. One such test using a drug called clomiphene may be able to predict your ability to ovulate up to twelve months into the future. The patient takes clomiphene pills for five days—from the fifth day after her period begins through day nine. Two weeks after she takes the last pill, the doctor draws blood and sends it to a lab to analyze the progesterone level in the blood. If the progesterone reaches a certain level, the patient will most likely continue to ovulate for at least one year. However, since we do not actually *see* an egg when we do this test, but make an assumption based on hormone levels, we cannot be absolutely certain that ovulation has occurred or will continue.

Right now, then, it's hard to tell exactly how long you'll

How to Enhance—and Stretch—Your Fertility

stay fertile. A lot depends on how healthy you are, your age, your family medical history, your genetic makeup—the list goes on and on. Your partner, too, is part of the equation. Even if you are fertile, together you may have difficulty conceiving.

Many women become pregnant later in life the natural way. For others, however, medical intervention is needed. For many years, Emily just couldn't decide whether or not she wanted to have a child, so it wasn't until she turned forty-three that she decided to take the plunge. She and her fifty-one-year-old husband, Seth, tried "naturally" for three months before consulting a fertility specialist, a colleague of mine in New York.

After putting Emily through a round of tests, including sonograms, blood tests, and cultures, they learned that she was in good shape, although her doctor suspected that she was no longer ovulating every month. But when Seth was tested, they discovered that although he had healthy sperm, it was deficient in numbers. They might eventually have a lucky break—or they might not. To hike their chances for successful conception with Seth's sperm, Emily's doctor recommended artificial insemination.

"We decided that we would try it for four months," Emily recalls. "After that we would stop, because I didn't want to have any surgery or to run the infertility gamut. That seemed too overwhelming. So to get things going and to overcome some of the problems, my doctor put me on clomiphene citrate [a drug to make you ovulate] and, later, HCG [human chorionic gonadotropin] shots to better time the inseminations with my ovulation. And guess what? I got pregnant on the first try!" At age forty-four, Emily gave birth to a healthy, nine-pound baby daughter.

Why It's Hard to Get Pregnant Later in Life

Emily's story points out two issues for transitional women: first, you *can* become pregnant and have a healthy baby when you're over thirty-five; and second, you may need to be willing to help Mother Nature along by taking advantage of today's newest technologies and methods. While navigable, the road to motherhood isn't always smooth or direct, particularly for women in their transitional years. Here's why.

Fewer—and older—eggs.

When you're born, your ovaries contain about a million cells, or potential ova. By the time you reach puberty, that number has already dwindled to about 400,000. Though that still seems like a lot, only about 300 to 500 might develop and ovulate as mature eggs—and that's the total number of fertilizable eggs your body will ever have. The numbers continue to decline as you get older; by the time you reach menopause, you have very few, if any, eggs left available for fertilization.

Additionally, the viability of your eggs drops as the years go by. An older egg is harder for a sperm to penetrate and is less receptive to a sperm that does get through.

The location of the eggs can also be a problem. Older eggs are more likely to be situated toward the middle of your ovary. In order for them to get to the periphery of the ovary where they can be released in ovulation, the eggs need to move through some scar tissue. Where does the scar tissue come from? The corpus luteum that forms each time you ovulate eventually degenerates, and in its place a mass of fibrous tissue, called the corpus albicans, is formed. In time, it, too, disappears—although it leaves behind a miniscule scar. The older you get, the more scar tissue you have and the more difficult it is for an older egg to reach the place on the ovary where it can be released and begin its journey to the fallopian tube.

Irregular ovulation.

Remember when we discussed why many transitional women suffer from changes or problems with their periods? You'll recall that one of the key reasons was that they may not be ovulating regularly. Well, this same problem can cause infertility. You can't get pregnant if you don't release a fertilizable egg.

Damage to reproductive organs.

The older you are, the greater the chances that you might have been exposed to an infection, such as chlamydia or some other sexually transmitted disease including gonorrhea or syphilis. An untreated STD can lead to pelvic inflammatory disease (PID), a catch-all term for infections that can adversely affect your fallopian tubes, ovaries, and/or uterus. PID can cause enough scarring to block your tubes and/or damage your ovaries, leaving you infertile.

Damage from gynecological surgeries.

Again, the older you are, the more likely it is that you've had gynecological surgeries that may have undermined your fertility. Obviously, the removal of an ovary due to cysts, hemorrhage, or infection lowers your chance for a successful pregnancy. However, even procedures that don't directly affect the ovaries can compromise your ability to conceive. The removal of uterine fibroids or other benign growths can cause adhesions, scar tissue that can obstruct your fallopian tubes and impede your eggs' natural, easy flow through the reproductive tract.

Health problems.

As you get older, your risk for such health problems as high blood pressure and kidney disease increases, and these ailments can reduce your chances for successful conception and pregnancy.

Male infertility.

Difficulty conceiving may also be due to the male partner, a subject I will discuss a little later on (see "Male Infertility," beginning on page 145).

How to Protect Your Fertility

If you plan to have a child in your transitional years, there are steps you can take to protect your fertility. For starters, here are a few things you can do.

Avoid sexually transmitted diseases (STDs).

Again, be aware that unless you detect an STD early and treat it aggressively with antibiotics, you may suffer irreparable damage to your reproductive organs.

Be alert for pelvic inflamatory disease (PID).

PID can be hard to detect, since symptoms range from an occasional dull ache around your belly to severe pain in your pelvis or abdomen. Other symptoms that may (but not always) appear include:

- *Nausea and vomiting.*
- *Lethargy or fatigue.*
- *Lower back pain.*
- *Burning or pain on urination.*
- *Foul-smelling vaginal discharge.*
- *Irregular bleeding or spotting.*
- *More, and more severe, menstrual cramps.*

Don't smoke.

A 1990 Report of the Surgeon General reveals that couples in which at least one partner smokes have a much higher rate of infertility than those in which both partners either have never smoked or have kicked the habit. The reason is that in women, smoking inhibits ovulation, reduces the number of eggs in the ovary, and interferes with the implantation of a fertilized egg within the uterus. It also raises the risk for ectopic pregnancy and miscarriage. In men, smoking appears to reduce the number of potent sperm cells in the ejaculate. If you're planning on having children, both you and your mate need to stop smoking—now!

Keep your ovaries healthy and intact.

To keep your ovaries in good working order, follow these three steps:

1. Have annual gynecological checkups that include an

internal pelvic exam. This is still the best way to detect signs of trouble early, while there's still time to treat any problem with as little disturbance to the ovaries as possible.

2. Call your doctor immediately if you notice any of the following:

- *A persistent dull or sharp ache* in your lower abdomen, which could signal PID, an ovarian cyst, or a twisted ovary.
- *Menstrual irregularities,* particularly mid-cycle spotting, which may indicate a benign or malignant tumor.
- *Mild but recurrent gastrointestinal upset,* which may indicate PID, or an enlarged ovary or ovarian cyst that is putting pressure on the bowel.
- *Increased urinary frequency,* which could signal a urinary tract infection.
- *Bloating or a sense of fullness* in your abdomen, which could indicate ovarian cysts, tumors, an enlarged ovary, or pelvic infection.

These symptoms aren't always a sign of a serious problem, but to be on the safe side, have your doctor check you out if you experience any of them.

3. Get a second opinion before agreeing to elective surgery on your ovaries. Stephanie, forty-two, came to see me after her family doctor had found a suspicious growth on her right ovary and had recommended surgery. Of course, she was panicked; in her mind, the growth had to mean cancer. But after doing a pelvic exam and an ultrasound, I believed that it was a harmless and quite common "functional" ovarian cyst, the kind that typically results from a slight hormonal imbalance during the menstrual cycle.

In Stephanie's case, the cyst was a greatly enlarged ovarian follicle that had failed to shrink normally. I suggested she wait two months to give the cyst a chance to disappear on its own. After two months, I saw that the growth was smaller, but still there. This time, I prescribed birth control pills to regulate Stephanie's cycle, thereby helping to shrink the cyst. Within weeks, it had disappeared for good—and all without ovarian surgery!

I am not opposed to all ovarian surgery, just unnecessary procedures. Sometimes surgery for certain abnormal growths is essential. If you have a tumor on your ovary, for example, and it appears to be growing very rapidly—and other tests strongly suggest a malignancy—then immediate surgery is the best option.

If your gynecologist suggests surgery for a noncancerous growth or cyst, ask if you could first try a noninvasive treatment, such as hormonal therapy. If surgery is necessary, explain that you'd like to keep as much of your ovary as possible. Many doctors assume that women forty or over aren't planning to have children and are not that concerned about losing an ovary. Whether or not you plan to have children, keep the ovary if you can. Often, the cyst or growth can be "shelled out" like a pea from a pod, leaving the healthy ovarian tissue essentially intact.

Exercise in moderation.

As I already mentioned in my ten-point plan in Chapter Two, if you work out too much, too hard, and too long, you may be undermining your fertility. Your best bet for good health: stick to a routine consisting of twenty to thirty minutes of sustained aerobic exercise three to four times a week. This will help protect your fertility and enhance your overall good health.

Watch your weight.

If you drop 10 to 14 percent below your proper weight, or climb 20 to 25 percent above it, you increase the chance that your brain will disrupt the sequence of hormonal events that normally leads to ovulation. Disturbing your hormonal balance can make miscarriage more likely. Of course, overweight and underweight women do get pregnant and give birth—so it's not a sure thing. To stay fertile for as long as possible and give yourself the best chance of carrying a baby to term, however, try to keep your weight at the optimal levels suggested in the weight chart on page 38.

Try not to get stressed out.

Trying to stay calmer and put problems and frustrations in perspective may help you conceive more easily and give birth successfully. While there's not a whole lot of hard-and-fast medical evidence that stress causes infertility, we do know that anxiety and tension can increase the production of opiates from the brain, and that these opiates can stop ovulation.

Many gynecologists, myself included, have observed that patients under a great deal of psychological stress are more likely to have a miscarriage than more relaxed moms-to-be. This may well be related to the fact that stress can raise your blood pressure and cause hypertension, a condition that we know increases the chances for miscarriage.

Another obvious link between stress and infertility centers on sexual desire. When you're very stressed out, you may feel too tired or too keyed up to have sex. As long as you're trying to conceive the natural way, this can be a big problem!

How to Enhance—and Stretch—Your Fertility

THE PREPREGNANCY CHECKUP

Once you decide you want to have a baby and you're over age thirty-five, it's best to take a fairly aggressive approach—and the older you are, the more aggressive I recommend you be. After all, at most a woman has only twelve opportunities—one a month—to get pregnant each year. Even if you've done your best to protect your fertility up until now, Mother Nature naturally limits the number of years in which even the healthiest transitional woman can conceive. If you're committed to having a baby, it's wise not to go about conception in a leisurely or haphazard manner—and from a medical point of view, that means undergoing a thorough physiological workup.

Your first step is to see your gynecologist. Since a successful pregnancy requires a strong, vital body, you need to have a general medical checkup, including an internal pelvic exam to help determine whether there's a problem with the size, shape, or position of your reproductive organs. You should also get a Pap smear to rule out cervical cancer, and a culture of your cervical secretions to see whether you have any problematic infections of which you were unaware.

Additionally, I recommend you get a urinalysis and blood studies, including a complete blood count and a health serum evaluation, which usually consists of about forty different blood tests that help scope out your general condition, including kidney function, cardiac and pulmonary condition, and blood sugar. It is also smart to get tested for rubella (German measles), hepatitis, and toxoplasmosis (the "cat box" disease) before trying to become pregnant, because contracting any of these diseases during pregnancy could lead to serious health problems with you or your fetus. If you've never had rubella or hepatitis, get vaccinated against them *now* because you'll have to wait about three more months before trying to get pregnant.

You're not the only one who needs to see a doctor, however. Your partner should have his testes, penis, and scrotum examined. He should also have a general physical, including a blood workup, to make sure that his and your blood types are compatible. Incompatible Rh factors or blood types can hurt your chances for conception and increase the likelihood of miscarriage. At this stage of the game, it's unlikely that your doctor will do a semen analysis.

Both of you should dig into your family medical backgrounds for any information that might affect your pregnancy or your baby. Tell your doctor if there is any family history of fetal loss, genetic abnormalities such as Down's syndrome, or sex-linked diseases such as hemophilia or muscular dystrophy. On the basis of this information you may choose to have chorionic villi sampling and/or amniocentesis during your pregnancy to make sure the fetus is developing properly. (Because these tests are well described in any number of pregnancy guidebooks, I have not covered them here. A simple visit to your local library or bookstore will provide you with all the information you need.)

Conceiving the Natural Way

Once your doctor has assured you that everything's A-OK, you're ready to try to conceive. The most effective and least expensive way to begin is to chart your basal body temperature. (To get started, see the basal body temperature chart on page 134.) Get a basal body oral thermometer (either the mercury type or one of the new digital models) that clearly measures in tenths of a degree. Then take your temperature for five minutes as soon as you wake up each morning—*before* getting out of bed, smoking, drinking, or eating. Record your reading by putting a dot on the chart at the intersection of the temperature and date lines. If your temperature is skewed by a fever or cold or any other cause, draw a line through that dot. Make sure to start a new chart the first day of your period and mark each day of menstruation by an *X*.

A woman's temperature is lower during the first part of the menstrual cycle than it is during the last part. About ten to twelve days into your cycle, you should notice your temperature drop and then rise abruptly the next morning by one half to one degree; this shows that you may be ovulating. Time your intercourse to coincide with your ovulation and indicate when you have intercourse with a circle. (Thus, you'll be circling the temperature dot.) If, after a month or two, you see that your temperature does not seem to vary—an indication that you may not be ovulating—tell your doctor. You may have a hormonal imbalance that can be treated easily.

If you find that taking your temperature each morning is too much of a chore, or if you just keep forgetting to do it, you might want to try an over-the-counter ovulation predictor kit, such as Clearplan Easy, First Response, Q-Test, Ovu Kit, Ovu Quick, or Answer. (Since all these tests are useful, I usually advise my patients to pick the one that is least expensive and/or most readily available.) By identifying when there is a rise in serum gonadotropin from the pituitary glands—the LH surge that occurs just prior to ovulation—these kits will let you know when you're ovulating. They do so with an indicator that changes color when dipped into your first morning urine.

If you're still not pregnant after having regular intercourse at the time of your ovulation for six months, waste

BASAL BODY TEMPERATURE CHART

Sample

Key: ● Marks daily body temperature
◉ Marks daily body temperature and intercourse
X Marks days of menstruation

How to Enhance—and Stretch—Your Fertility

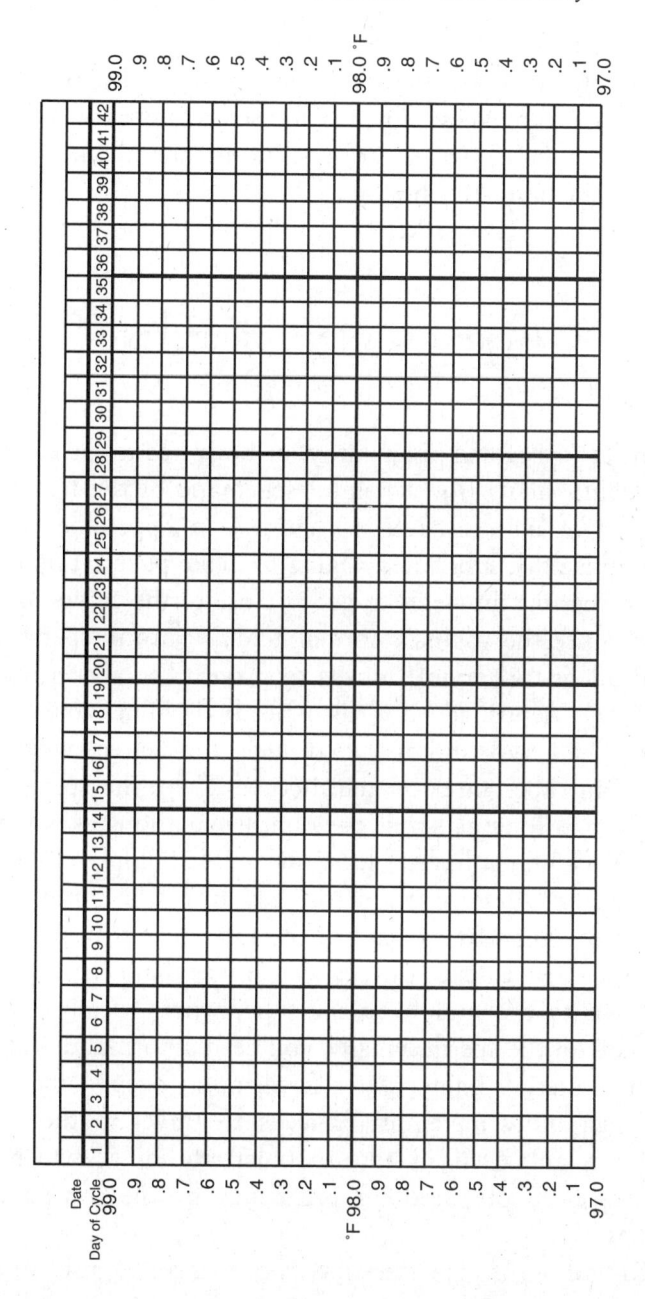

no time finding out what additional steps you might take, preferably with the help of a fertility specialist. Because it takes two to make a baby, I will discuss infertility problems and solutions in two separate sections: one about you and one about him. You first.

Checking—and Correcting—Your Anatomy

In order to become pregnant, your body has to have certain key components (for a helpful schematic of the female reproductive anatomy, refer to figure A in Appendix A). You need a healthy, lubricated vagina to make penetration easier and to permit the penis to get as close to the cervix as possible. Since the vagina's normal acidity can kill sperm, you need adequate cervical mucus to protect the sperm once it has been deposited. You also need "holding zones" just above the cervix and at the *cornuae* (those areas where the fallopian tubes meet on the uterus). There the sperm may stay for as long as seven days until ovulation takes place.

You also must have at least one viable fallopian tube that is open and able to admit the egg from the *fimbria*—the "catcher's mitt" at the end of the tube near the ovary. The fimbria safely catches the egg as it leaves the ovary and rolls it down to the middle of the tube, where ideally the egg meets with the sperm. Finally, you need a normal uterus and healthy uterine lining. After fertilization occurs, the fertilized egg (now an embryo) needs to travel to the uterus and implant itself in the endometrial lining, which has already been prepared for pregnancy by the ovarian hormones.

To find out if your infertility is due to some problem with

your pelvic anatomy, you'll probably undergo one or more of the following tests:

Postcoital or Huhner's Test.

One of the first-line ways to diagnose an anatomical problem—specifically, whether the sperm can survive your cervical mucus—is a postcoital test. It should be done just prior to ovulation, since only preovulatory mucus will allow the sperm to remain active and potent. You will be asked to have intercourse with your mate either the night before or the morning of the test. Then you'll go to your doctor's office, where he or she will obtain a sample of your cervical mucus to see if there are enough active sperm to do the job. Inhospitable cervical mucus will fail to protect the sperm, which will be killed off before conception can occur.

Hysterosalpingogram (HSG).

With an HSG, a procedure that is usually performed in the radiology department of your hospital, a contrast, or dye, is inserted through your cervix. While watching the dye's progress through the uterus and out the fallopian tubes on a fluoroscopic video scanner, your doctor can see any abnormalities in the cervix, the inside of your uterus, or your tubes, and can also see how your tubes empty.

You don't need to do anything to prepare for this test, although the doctor will want to know if you have any allergies, especially to such foods as shellfish, since there is iodine in the dye. Although some patients complain of cramping during the injection of the contrast and for several hours afterward, I can't give any strong painkillers or tranquilizers for this test. The reason is that I need to see if your uterus begins to spasm as the dye goes to the fallopian tubes. If it does, it indicates that your uterus may also spasm in intercourse as the sperm goes to the fallopian tubes, which can inhibit fertility. Giving you any drugs would relax the uterus and could disguise this problem.

Diagnostic laparoscopy.

Since the HSG can miss adhesions or scar tissue located around the fimbria or on the outside of the tubes, your doctor may do a diagnostic laparoscopy. In order to get a better look at your uterus, tubes, and ovaries, he or she inserts a lighted tubelike instrument called a laparoscope (a fiberoptic instrument) into your abdomen through a small incision made below the navel. Usually, a video camera is placed on the laparoscope so that your organs can be seen on a video screen. Sometimes a video is taped for later study. Again, contrast is injected through the cervix to be sure the tubes are open. While laparoscopy is helpful, because it reveals a good deal of information, it is not to be undergone lightly, since it involves general anesthesia.

Hysteroscopy.

Usually done at the same time as a laparoscopy, the hysteroscopy involves inserting a small, telescopelike instrument through the vagina and cervix into your uterus so that your doctor can get an additional look at the uterine lining and the openings of the fallopian tubes and check for tumors or adhesions. The doctor also can confirm or rule out any suspicion of submucous fibroids, or such congenital abnormalities as a uterine septum (a wall of tissue dividing the uterus in two) or a double uterus, any of which could hinder conception.

Falloposcopy.

This new procedure is like a superhysteroscopy. It allows the doctor to follow the tubes from within the uterus out farther, toward the fimbria. It usually requires general anesthesia, though under certain circumstances local anesthetics can be used. Falloposcopy isn't done very often, since 90 percent of the time the other procedures usually suffice.

How to Fix an Anatomical Problem

Let's suppose one of these diagnostic tests reveals an anatomical problem. If it's not too severe, your doctor may be able to correct it during the diagnostic procedure itself.

Say, for example, that your doctor finds evidence of mild or moderate endometriosis, a condition in which the same type of tissue that usually lines the endometrium grows in or on other parts of the body. Or suppose there are adhesions, scarring, or any other abnormality on the outside of your tubes, uterus, or ovaries that is discovered during the laparoscopy. These problems can be treated by operating through the laparoscope at the time the diagnostic procedure is performed. If problems exist inside the uterus or tubes, a hysteroscope or falloposcope can be used to remove scar tissue, polyps, or fibroids, although such surgery requires general anesthesia.

One of these procedures helped Jamie, thirty-eight, and her husband, Peter, forty-six, fulfill their desire to have a child. Jamie came to see me a few years ago, soon after she'd married. She and Peter had been trying to get pregnant for six months using the basal body temperature method, but without any success. When I took Jamie's medical history, I learned she'd long had problems with menstrual irregularity. For a while, birth control pills had corrected this problem, but now that she'd been off the Pill for nine months, the irregularity had returned.

Initial steps to check the couple's fertility didn't reveal much. Peter's semen analysis showed normal sperm with satisfactory movement and numbers; Jamie's endometrial biopsy showed she was ovulating. However, when we did a hysterosalpingogram (HSG), we identified a problem. The test suggested that Jamie's fallopian tubes might be blocked, since there was no spillage of dye out of either tube.

Next, I suggested that we do a laparoscopy. I explained to Jamie that if this test confirmed that her tubes were blocked, we would try to use laser or microsurgery at the same time to correct any defect. And that's precisely what we did: we found blockage from adhesions in both tubes and used a laser technique to open them.

It took Jamie about three months to heal. During this time, she and her husband made no attempts to become pregnant. Then I put her on medication, clomiphene citrate, to regulate her ovulations. After six months, she became pregnant. Nine months later, Jamie gave birth to a healthy baby boy.

As I'm sure Jamie would agree, the fact that doctors can correct many problems with laser, cautery (using heat to burn away undesirable tissue), or microsurgery through the laparoscope is a tremendous boon for couples trying to become pregnant. Only ten years ago, women whose infertility was caused by anatomical problems had no choice but to undergo general surgery to clear adhesions, destroy endometrial implants (tissue from the endometrium that is found in an area of the pelvis where it doesn't belong), correct scars from endometriosis, clear fallopian tubes, or remove abnormal lesions of the uterus. In contrast, the new procedures don't leave a large incision scar, don't expose the bowel—which means you're up and about *much* quicker—and result in few if any complications or side effects.

If any of these procedures reveals a serious need for further surgery—for instance, if a large portion of your fallopian tube is abnormal or tests show a large fibroid or tumor—your doctor may recommend a laparotomy; that is, traditional abdominal surgery. But since laparotomy itself can cause adhesions and scarring, and since recuperation is usually fairly slow and difficult, doctors don't like to do it unless it is absolutely necessary. Many times patients are referred for assisted reproductive technologies (ART) rather than undergoing the intensive surgical procedures. (I'll discuss ART later in this chapter.)

Checking—and Correcting— Your Cycles

Let's say your anatomy is in pretty good shape. In that case, the reason you're having trouble getting pregnant may be one of three functional problems:

1. The follicles within your ovary are not growing properly.
2. You're not ovulating.
3. The lining of your uterus is not adequately preparing for the presence of an embryo.

There are several ways to see if you are ovulating.

1. *Take your basal body temperature each morning.* Do this as I described earlier. If after a few months you find

your temperature remains constant, it may signal that you're not ovulating.

2. *During these same few months, use an over-the-counter ovulation test kit.* (I've named some of the most popular on page 133.) If the results are always negative, that's another sign that you may not be ovulating.

3. *Have serial ultrasound.* Your doctor may suggest having an ultrasound test of your ovaries every two or three days during the first half of your cycle to see if the follicles are developing properly. If they aren't, you may not be producing eggs to fertilize.

4. *Have your progesterone level tested.* If you've ovulated, your progesterone will rise to a certain level. Your doctor may also want to run a few other hormonal studies to see if your LH, FSH, and estradiol (estrogen) levels are satisfactory.

5. *Undergo endometrial sampling.* In a quick office procedure, your doctor will take a sample of the tissue of your endometrium, usually on the twenty-second day of your twenty-eight day cycle; by examining the tissue he or she will be able to tell whether or when you're ovulating.

Endometrial sampling will also reveal whether you've got a functional problem with your uterus. For example, it could show that the lining is not responding properly to your hormones, which means that it isn't being readied to receive the embryo. Depending on the cause of the problem, the condition may be treated with surgery or hormones.

How to Enhance—and Stretch—Your Fertility

Using fertility drugs to fix functional problems.

When there's something askew with what we call your hormonal "milieu"—that is, your body's hormonal environment—hormone therapy may allow you and your partner to achieve a healthy pregnancy.

FERTILITY DRUGS. Let's suppose you've got an ovulation problem. In that case, the best course of treatment is medications that will trigger ovulation. Among the most widely prescribed are:

• *Clomiphene citrate.* Known by the brand names Clomid and Serophene, this drug is actually a weak estrogen that acts to fool your pituitary gland into secreting increased amounts of gonadotropins, which brings about ovulation. You generally take it orally for five days, from the fifth to ninth day of your cycle.

• *Human chorionic gonadotropin (HCG).* HCG is injected once at mid-cycle to induce ovulation by stimulating the LH surge. Often, HCG is given with clomiphene citrate (above).

• *Menotropins.* Menotropins consist of a combination of FSH and LH. These hormones promote growth and development of the follicle of the ovary. When such menotropins as Pergonal (LH and FSH) and Metrodin (FSH only) are used, HCG is also given to stimulate ovulation. You get injections of the menotropins daily in carefully calculated doses until mid-cycle, when HCG is added.

• *Gonadotropin-releasing hormone (GnRH).* Known by the synthetic brand names Lupron and Synerel, this hormone is injected when natural GnRH is inadequate or completely absent. The drug Lutrepluse is released at biologically correct intervals from a small, timed, battery-operated mechanism that you wear. This controls your pituitary and triggers ovulation.

- *Bromergocryptine.* This drug, known by its brand name, Parlodel, acts to restore ovulation and a regular cycle in women who show elevated prolactin levels. An increased level of prolactin can cause you to stop ovulating and bring about abnormal lactation (the release of milk from the breast).

The downside of fertility drugs.

As always, drug treatments have their drawbacks. With fertility drugs, there are three:

1. Multiple births. Fertility drugs usually stimulate the ovary to prepare and eject an egg. Sometimes they overdo it and hyperstimulate the ovary, which releases several eggs. This can result in multiple fetuses, which means you may give birth to triplets, quadruplets, quintuplets, or more. Multiple births are much riskier for the mother because they increase her chances for hypertension, preeclampsia (toxemia of pregnancy that could lead to convulsive seizures, induced labor, cesarean section, or even coma during pregnancy), and premature delivery.

Multiple births are more risky for the babies because they're often born prematurely. Multiple birth babies also have a greater chance of suffering from various abnormalities. A recent University of South Florida study of over 1,200 twin pregnancies, for example, showed that the risk for abnormalities is twice as high for twins as for single birth babies.

If your doctor detects the possibility of multiple births very early on, he or she may be able to remove some of the fertilized eggs at that time, but this is a recent innovation and is neither always successful nor always desired.

2. *Higher risk for ovarian cancer.* An epidemiologic survey conducted by scientists at Stanford University and published in 1992 found that infertile women who were treated with fertility drugs and still failed to get pregnant had a higher risk for ovarian cancer later on in life. Understand, however, that there is a good deal of argument over this data because other scientists feel there were too many variables in the study that were not controlled for—for example, patients took different drugs for different periods of time. Now, both the National Institutes of Health and the National Cancer Institute are providing funds for additional study so that more definite conclusions can be drawn. Unfortunately, it will take some time before we get a final answer.

3. *Time and money.* It takes a lot of time and energy to take fertility drugs properly and to undergo the necessary medical workups and follow-through. What's more, these drugs are expensive and aren't always covered by insurance.

Male Infertility

What you've heard is true: men do remain fertile longer than women. A healthy man can father a child well into his fifties, probably into his sixties, and occasionally even beyond. But when a couple finds they're having a problem getting pregnant, some 50 to 55 percent of the time it's due to a problem with the male. If you've been trying for a few months with no luck, it's important that your partner get checked out before you get heavily involved with further procedures yourself.

The first step is to do semen analyses, studies of the fresh ejaculate, which consists of sperm and seminal fluid. Since sperm levels differ from day to day, three separate semen analyses taken on three separate days are needed to determine whether there is enough semen being ejaculated and whether it has sufficient sperm. The sperm are evaluated for number (called sperm count, or density), the percentage that are moving, the quality of the forward movement (or progression), and morphology (shape and form.) Trouble in any of these departments may explain why you're not getting pregnant easily.

If the semen analyses reveal a more serious difficulty, such as abnormal sperm or no sperm, additional tests must be done to find the source of the problem. These may include testes biopsies, X-ray vasography, prostate ultrasound, magnetic resonance imaging (MRI), thermography, venography (injecting a dye into the spermatic vein), and ultrasound of the vesicles in the ducts. (See figure 3 on page 117 for a diagram of the male reproductive anatomy.)

Before you undertake advanced tests, see if you can rule out any possible simple reasons for your partner's infertility. Because sperm production takes three months, any injury to the sperm in the three months prior to testing could weaken its potency. Sperm damage can result from any one of the following:

Hot tubs.

Taking a turn in a hot tub may be relaxing, but the excess heat on testicles causes a decrease in sperm production. Steam rooms and Jacuzzis can have a similar effect.

Tight underwear or athletic supporters.

Overly snug undergarments can also overheat the testes. This is often a problem among professional athletes and amateur "jocks" and explains why boxer shorts are popular with fathers-to-be.

Untreated venereal disease.

If your partner was ever exposed to venereal disease and did not seek treatment, he may not have enough or sufficiently potent sperm. Additionally, adhesions caused by these infections could have damaged his tubes (the vas deferens and ejaculatory duct) and prevent delivery of the semen.

Lubrications used during intercourse.

Sometimes, seemingly innocent over-the-counter lubricants (for example, K-Y Jelly) can be toxic to sperm and reduce male fertility.

Frequent intercourse.

Having intercourse more than twice a day can be counterproductive. In their zeal to try to "make a baby," couples sometimes have intercourse several times a day. This approach actually works against successful fertilization because after two or so ejaculations, the sperm count in the ejaculate drops too low to be effective. In order for the man to have enough time to store up more, and more potent, sperm, it's best to limit intercourse to every other day.

Medications, medical treatments, and street drugs.

Medications such as cortisone, colchicine, and antileukemic drugs—as well as medical treatments such as radiation therapy—can be harmful to sperm and gonads. Street drugs, including marijuana and crack/cocaine, can also cause problems, including reducing the growth of sperm, decreasing or toxifying seminal fluid (the fluid from the prostate and seminal ducts in which we find spermatozoa), or triggering spasms of the seminal ducts, which can prevent ejaculation.

More complicated causes of male infertility include:

Hormonal problems.

Sperm need certain hormones, specifically FSH and LH, in order to grow and develop. If your partner's hormonal milieu is out of kilter, this can prevent adequate or regular release of FSH and LH. The result: infertility. Such hormonal difficulties can be detected by determining FSH, LH, and testosterone levels in the blood.

A bad semen/cervical mucus reaction.

A problem can arise if your partner's semen and your cervical mucus react against each other. If your mucus has antibodies to your partner's sperm, these antibodies can stun the sperm that enter the vagina or cause the sperm to clump together so that they cannot move or react. Fortunately, this predicament is rare and can be overcome. Artificial insemination allows the sperm to bypass contact with the cervical mucus and go directly to the safe holding areas in the tubes. Medication or other treatments to the sperm can also be helpful.

How to Correct Male Infertility

If the problem is related to life-style or habits, some simple changes in behavior—avoiding long soaks in a hot tub, wearing loose underwear, steering clear of drugs—often do the trick. But if the problem is anatomical or hormonal, more aggressive steps must be taken.

Surgical remedies.

When there's an anatomical difficulty, such as adhesions or abnormal blood vessels or ducts, surgery can be a welcome remedy. The most widespread procedure is the removal of a *varicocele*, a dilated blood vessel in the scrotum that reduces both sperm count and sperm activity. This procedure is usually done under general anesthesia, although a local anesthetic may be used at some medical centers. Other surgical procedures can also help to clear tubes, particularly the vas deferens and ejaculatory duct, and correct adhesions.

Hormone therapy.

When the problem is hormonal, treatment is, unfortunately, quite limited. That's because male reproduction is not cyclic, like the female's. To treat a male fertility problem, you would need to have constant high dosage hormonal therapy, which is medically unwise, since it can make the testes dangerously hyperactive. By contrast, female infertility can be treated by very low doses of hormones that are given for short periods of time. However, there are still a few male-oriented tactics to try.

If your partner's gonadotropins FSH and LH are low, daily injections of HCG (high LH) might help, since LH is essential for successful growth and development of the sperm. Pergonal (consisting of LH and FSH) can also be injected in small daily doses, though the improvement rate isn't very high. Some doctors might recommend clomiphene citrate and testosterone, but most specialists doubt the effectiveness of these drugs.

High-Tech Solutions to Infertility Problems

Some infertility problems, whether male or female, anatomical or hormonal, can't be corrected to the point that you and your mate can get pregnant on your own. Yet there's still hope. The medical community has come a long way in helping you surmount your problems and achieve a successful pregnancy.

Artificial insemination.

When you're in great shape but your partner's sperm is less than ideal, artificial insemination is often a good bet. You can use your partner's sperm even if it has reduced numbers or activity because artificial insemination enhances the sperm's viability by placing it right into the cervical mucus or uterus where it has a better chance of reaching an egg. This procedure is called Artificial Insemination Homologous (AIH).

If your mate has inactive sperm or no sperm at all, you'll need to have donor insemination with sperm supplied by a sperm bank. This procedure is called Artificial Insemination Donor (AID). These days, sperm banks offer you as much information about each donor as possible so that you can choose one who resembles your real partner. There's even a bank in California where you can get the sperm of Nobel Prize winners!

Much more important, however, is to find a bank that meticulously screens for HIV virus, hepatitis, and other significant diseases, such as Tay-Sachs and sickle-cell anemia. Unfortunately, sperm banks are not federally controlled, and to date, only a few states, including New York and California, have issued any regulations for screening procedures at all. To find out about the status of sperm banks in your state, call your local health department. If you live in a state with nonregulated banks, you'll pretty much have to go on faith. The American Fertility Society in Birmingham, Alabama, will send you a printout of sperm banks, but it does not inspect or screen them.

You could—and should—ask your gynecologist or fertility specialist to recommend a particular bank. I'd also urge you to find a bank that's been around for at least ten years. Since a single serious slipup (such as selling sperm from an HIV-infected donor) can close a sperm bank quickly, those in business for a long time are probably a safer bet.

Once you have found a sperm source, your doctor will probably suggest one of two techniques, depending upon the source and condition of the sperm: ICI (intracervical insemination) or IUI (intrauterine insemination).

INTRACERVICAL INSEMINATION (ICI). With this procedure, your doctor uses a special syringe to place the sperm into your vagina at the cervix, just where it is deposited in sexual intercourse. This procedure is very quick, but you will need to remain on the examination table with your feet in the stirrups for twenty minutes. Another possible option is to put sperm into a cervical cap, which is then placed over your cervix and left inside you for two to four hours.

INTRAUTERINE INSEMINATION (IUI). When there's less-than-desirable sperm, or when the cervix or its mucus is abnormal or antagonistic to the sperm, intrauterine insemination is the preferred approach. In this procedure, the sperm is first prepared by centrifuging it into a pellet. Then the pellet is placed into a special, sterile "capacitating" solution that makes the sperm more capable of fertilization. The resulting mixture is then inserted through your cervix and into the uterus.

The American Fertility Society says that if there aren't any problems with the woman's reproductive tract, the success rate for insemination with a donor should equal that of normal conception. Your chances of successfully conceiving with artificial insemination depend on a variety of additional factors, from your own hormone levels to the condition of the sperm used.

Artificial insemination has only a couple of drawbacks. Uterine infection can occur with IUI, but it's rare. The procedure also can be a bit pricey. While each insemination isn't that costly—no more than $200 per try—at about two tries per month, the bill can mount up quickly. Sometimes insurance will cover the procedures, but not always, so be sure to check your policy carefully.

Higher tech options.

If artificial insemination doesn't work for you, you still have a few options available, thanks to assisted reproductive technologies (ART). Although each procedure is slightly different, the basic method is the same: eggs are removed from your body taken to a certain degree of maturation in a Petri dish and inseminated before being put back into a uterus to grow and develop into a (hopefully) normal, healthy baby. You've probably read about some of these modern miracles already, but here's a quick run-through.

How to Enhance—and Stretch—Your Fertility

IN VITRO FERTILIZATION (IVF). We use IVF most often on women whose ovaries and uterus are in good shape but whose fallopian tubes are not. Each year, some 20,000 couples undergo IVF. Since the first "test tube baby" some fourteen years ago, more than 10,000 IVF babies have been born in the United States. These statistics are not all that favorable, because IVF is not always successful, and even when pregnancy does occur, the early miscarriage rate is high. According to the American Fertility Society, the delivery rate for IVF is about 15 percent.

With IVF, we extract mature eggs from your ovary and then fertilize them outside of your body in a Petri dish. Sounds simple, right? Not quite. The procedure actually involves several technical steps.

First, your doctor will give you Pergonal to help lots of follicles start growing so that you'll have a greater pool of mature eggs with which to work. The growth of the eggs is monitored by ultrasound. Next, at mid-cycle as many eggs as possible are removed (or "harvested") from your ovary. This can be done through the vagina using a local anesthetic, or with a laparoscope using general anesthetic. (The first method is preferable, since you can avoid the risks involved with general anesthesia.) Once the eggs are removed, a few are used and the rest are frozen and stored as backup.

Next, the fresh eggs are fertilized by sperm—if possible, your partner's—in a Petri dish and placed in an incubator, where they are permitted to form an embryo, for about two days. Since the ovarian hormones have already prepared your endometrium to receive an embryo, several embryos are then inserted through your cervix and into the endometrium. With any luck, they'll embed there and nature will take its course.

If you've undergone premature menopause, or if for genetic reasons it isn't wise for you to become pregnant with your own eggs, you could be a candidate for a variation of IVF called *donor egg IVF*. Here, another woman—your donor—goes through the first several steps of the process. Then, when the embryo is ready to be transferred back into the body, it goes into *your* body. The mother's cycle is synchronized with the donor's by giving the mother estrogen and progesterone therapy.

There are some sticky legal issues involved in donor egg IVF, most of which center on who is the biological mother. So before going through this procedure, it's a good idea to speak with a lawyer experienced in these matters.

GAMETE INTRAFALLOPIAN TRANSFER (GIFT). Basically, GIFT follows the same steps as IVF, but there are three significant differences. First, the harvested eggs are mixed with sperm that have been enhanced to make them more capable of fertilization in a process similar to how sperm are prepared for IVF. Second, this mixture—not just the embryos—is returned to the body. And third, the mixture is transferred by laparoscopy into the fallopian tubes. Putting this mixture into the tubes closely mimics the pattern of normal biological conception, which is why it works so well.

GIFT has a higher success rate than IVF. According to the American Fertility Society, 26.6 percent of GIFT patients have a live delivery. In order for GIFT to work, however, you must have at least one healthy, open tube. If your tubes are scarred or missing, GIFT isn't for you.

ZYGOTE INTRAFALLOPIAN TRANSFER (ZIFT). ZIFT involves the same basic procedure as GIFT, but actual embryos—not the egg-and-sperm mixture—are inserted into the fallopian tube. In order to be a good candidate for ZIFT, you need to have at least enough healthy tube for insertion of the embryo. The delivery rate for ZIFT is 19.7 percent. It is lower than GIFT because you are working with an older embryo that may have passed the time when it could successfully implant into the uterine wall; frequently, the uterus rejects the embryo as it would any foreign body.

ZONA DRILLING. There's one more assisted technique—so new that it's only in the testing stage—that I want to mention: zona drilling. Scientists theorize that if fertilization is not occurring in the early stages of IVF, it may be because the sperm isn't able to penetrate the egg. With zona drilling, an opening is made in the *zona pellucida*, the thick membranous envelope surrounding the egg, to help the sperm enter more easily. Since this technique is only in its experimental phase, there are no data as to its success.

The downside of higher tech procedures.

As terrific as assisted reproductive technologies are, they are not without some liabilities. The procedures are expensive, costing anywhere from $8,000 to $10,000 or more depending on what part of the country you're in, and insurance doesn't always cover the expense. Also, as with any pregnancy, there's a chance of miscarriage or even ectopic pregnancy.

Additionally, because you're given Pergonal first, you have the same risks and possible side effects involved in any hormonal treatments. Moreover, with IVF there's an increased chance for risky multiple births. But despite these drawbacks, fertility technology has given new hope to couples who could otherwise have never had their own babies.

When You Can't Give Birth to Your Own Baby

These miracles of modern reproductive technology are offering new hope to thousands of transitional women, and that's great. But at some point, you may have to face the fact that you're not going to be able to give birth to your own baby.

I wish I could offer you some sage advice as to when you should call it quits, but I can't. This is a highly personal decision that only you and your partner can make. Some of my patients have been incredibly persistent and ultimately successful. Others who were just as determined were not so lucky. I've found it helps to ask yourselves these questions every now and then and answer them as honestly as possible:

- *Why do we really want to have a child?*
- *Does it have to be our biological child?*
- *What need would giving birth fulfill?*
- *How important is fulfilling that need to our emotional and physical health?*
- *What does having a baby mean to our marriage?*
- *What does having a baby mean to our position in our extended family and in our community of friends and neighbors?*

Grappling with these issues may help you know when it's right to stop and when or if you can consider other ways to bring a child into your life, such as surrogacy, adoption, even becoming foster parents. Space constraints don't permit me to discuss these methods in much detail, and it's really not necessary since one trip to your local library or bookstore will offer reams of helpful material on each.

My best advice is this: while pregnancy and childbirth are some of life's best experiences, they're just one small part of being a mother. Nurturing a child, teaching him or her how the world works, passing along your values, taking care of him when he's sick, and comforting him when he's frightened or upset are what make you a parent, what make you a "real" mom. Giving birth is only one way to begin.

7

How to Enjoy the Best Sex Ever

- Physical Problems that Can Interfere with Intimacy
- Gynecological Abnormalities
- Gynecological Surgeries
- Chronic Illness
- Endometriosis
- The Effect of Medications
- When the Problem Is Emotional
- Strategies to Spice Up Your Sex Life
- Men's Sexual Problems
- Help for Men

Transitional women often find themselves in a sexual predicament. On the one hand, they have the physical ability to become aroused more quickly than ever. Many have greater and more readily occurring orgasms than they did when they were in their twenties. Emotional maturity also adds to their sexual potential. Most transitional women feel much more confident in themselves and more secure about who they are and what they want than they felt when they were younger. Thus, they can be less shy about initiating contact and expressing their sexual needs and desires.

On the other hand, there's this undeniable and perplexing fact: many transitional women seem to lose their desire for sex. Carole, a thirty-eight-year-old systems analyst and mother of two teenagers, is one of my patients who raised this subject during her six-month checkup.

"Bernie, I'm confused," said Carole. "I used to love sex. And I still enjoy making love with my husband. But, well, I'm just not that *interested*. It's as if I've lost my sex drive. It's really causing problems in my marriage, not just because my husband's sex drive is still strong, but because he thinks I don't love him anymore. It's not true; after sixteen years of marriage, I love him more than ever. I find him attractive, but I just don't seem to have the same desire. What's happened to me?"

Physical Problems that Can Interfere with Intimacy

A healthy woman in her transitional years can expect to enjoy good sex for a long, long time. However, some physical problems tend to crop up during the transitional years that can put a damper on sexual desire. Women who experience any number of conditions, from vaginal dryness to fibroids or other tumors in the pelvic area, may truly feel pain or discomfort during sex. It's not surprising, then, that their desire for sexual intimacy may plummet. If you think a physical problem may be interfering with your sex life, read on.

Vaginal dryness.

In order to explain why your vagina may be drier, let's run through a quick lesson on one aspect of Masters' and Johnson's sex research. Their work suggests that pleasurable intercourse has four stages:

1. The excitement stage, during which stimulation of the erogenous zones or erotic fantasizing causes you to become aroused. (In transitional women the veins in the genital area become more rapidly engorged during sexual contact, which sparks intense excitement.)
2. The plateau stage, when physical stimulation brings about a sustained level of excitement.
3. The orgasmic stage, in which excitement peaks.
4. The resolution stage, during which the body relaxes, and other changes, such as increased sweating or hyperventilation, gradually diminish.

A young woman's vagina is easily and quickly lubricated during the excitement stage, thanks to the plentiful secretions of the vaginal walls. This lubrication prepares the vagina for easy, comfortable penetration. A transitional woman, particularly after age forty, may find she has slightly less abundant secretions at the opening of the vagina during that stage, making penetration less comfortable. As she reaches forty-five and beyond, she is much more likely to experience vaginal dryness and its accompanying discomfort.

When the *external* portion of your vagina/vulva stays dry during sexual activity, the problem is usually hormonal. Because your ovaries are less able to change androgen into estrogen after age thirty-five, androgen levels are likely to increase in the transitional years. Androgen has been linked with sexual appetite, so greater levels of this hormone should, at least theoretically, enhance your sexual desire.

Yet the powerful effect of decreasing estrogen—which may cause vaginal dryness and reduce vaginal turgor, making penetration more difficult and less satisfying—is greater than the impact of increasing androgens. Your libidinal balance, therefore, tips in favor of pain rather than pleasure; you might feel sexy, but not comfortable during intercourse.

When the *internal* portion of your vagina stays dry, hormones are not at fault. In that case, the problem is usually psychosexual; for some emotional reason, you are not getting aroused, a problem which we'll discuss shortly.

Vaginal atrophy.

By the time you've reached the latter part of your transitional years—ages forty-five to fifty—your vaginal walls will begin to thin and shrink. (For a useful view of your reproductive anatomy, see figure 4.) When the walls of the vagina become thinner, they don't cushion the nearby urethra and bladder as well during intercourse, which can make sex uncomfortable. The mons and labia also may begin to lose their fatty padding, which can lead to less enjoyable intercourse.

Keeping the vagina in good shape.

Sexual problems caused by a dry vagina or vaginal atrophy can be alleviated in several ways.

- *An over-the-counter lubricant or moisturizer.* Buy a pure lipid lubricant like K-Y Jelly or H-R Jelly at your local drugstore and apply it to the vulvar region and partway into the vagina just before having intercourse. It should make penetration much more comfortable.

FIGURE 4. *Side View of Female Reproductive Anatomy*

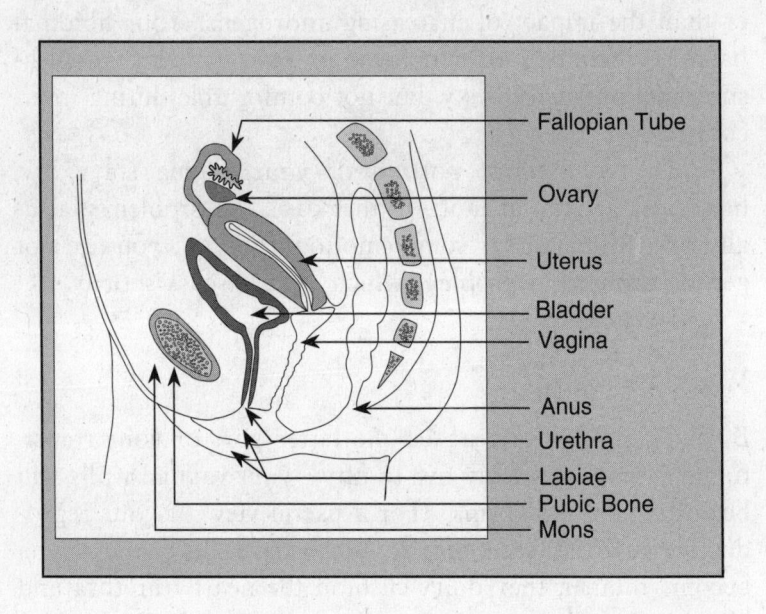

- Fallopian Tube
- Ovary
- Uterus
- Bladder
- Vagina
- Anus
- Urethra
- Labiae
- Pubic Bone
- Mons

If you want a longer-lasting, though more expensive, product, you can try Replens, a vaginal moisturizer with a consistency more like hand lotion than lubricating jelly. Its "bioadhesive properties" make it stick to the mucous membranes of the vagina, which is why it lasts longer than the jellies.

• *Vaginal suppositories.* If the above lubricants don't work, suppositories might help. The brand that I often recommend is Lubrin, unscented inserts that liquefy inside the vagina and simulate natural lubrication. The effect usually lasts for several hours.

• *Estrogen.* If you can take it safely, estrogen supplementation will help get your vagina in shape. If you don't want to take pills, an estrogen cream or gel applied locally once or twice a week (depending upon the individual) will also improve the vagina and labia by helping to increase turgor and offering lubrication.

- *Kegel exercises.* If you've ever had a vaginal delivery, you probably know all about Kegel exercises. If not, here's what you do: concentrate on your vagina and try to move it repeatedly. (Some people liken this exercise to an elevator making stops at different floors.) It takes some practice but you'll soon get the hang of it. Doing Kegels regularly exercises the muscles that lie under the mucous membranes of the vagina. This helps bring blood and oxygen to the area and keeps your vagina toned up.
- *Masturbation.* When you masturbate, you actually go through all the stages of the sexual act. Regular masturbation helps keep the nerves and muscles of the vagina primed and ready.

Gynecological Abnormalities

Vaginal dryness and atrophy aren't abnormalities; they're age-related problems that nearly all transitional women experience at some point. But there are other physical difficulties that can occur at any time, although they do tend to appear more frequently in the transitional years. If left untreated, they, too, can prevent you from fulfilling your sexual promise. These problems fall under the category of "gynecological abnormalities."

Fibroids.

Fibroids (myomas), which are fairly common in transitional women—some 60 percent have them—are benign tumors found in the uterus. They're situated either on top of the uterine muscles, within the muscles themselves, or underneath the lining of the uterus. In most cases, the patient won't know they're there, but during an internal gynecological exam, your doctor may feel a hardness in your uterus. If fibroids develop near the cervix and press on surrounding nerves, however, you will probably feel persistent pain. Occasionally, fibroids grow so large that they dramatically distort the uterus, forcing it to impinge upon the vagina. As a result, sexual penetration can be difficult and uncomfortable.

Some fibroids can cause excessive vaginal bleeding during your period. The reason is that these growths prevent the uterus from clamping down properly at the end of your cycle. In fact, excessive menstrual bleeding may be the symptom that tips your doctor off to the presence of fibroids that he or she may not even be able to feel; in that case, he or she will probably do an endometrial biopsy, or D&C and ultrasound of the pelvic area, to confirm whether or not fibroids are present and where they are.

Some fibroids can be reduced with the help of such antiestrogen drugs as Lupron, which is injected into the muscle of your arm or buttocks, and Synerol, which is sniffed. But since these medications work against estrogen in your system, they bring on some menopausal symptoms, such as a dry vagina. Additionally, fibroids can return once medication is stopped.

If fibroids are excessively large or numerous, the most effective treatment that will allow you to keep your uterus is a myomectomy, the surgical removal of the fibroids through the abdomen. Unfortunately, fibroids are stubborn and can return even after myomectomy. Sometimes, a hysterectomy is necessary.

Infections.

Gynecological infections can occur at just about any age, since they have more to do with sexual frequency and activity (including the number of sexual partners) than with how old you are. Local infections of the vagina or cervix can cause vaginal discharges that can stain your clothes and carry an unpleasant odor, making sex both embarrassing and unpleasant. They can also irritate your vagina and make lovemaking uncomfortable. Infections involving the fallopian tubes and ovaries may result in abscesses or adhesions that can cause abdominal and pelvic pain—another sexual turnoff. Among the most widespread infections are:

YEAST INFECTIONS. Vaginal yeast infections often occur in transitional women. In part, that's because over the years their vaginas have been exposed to a variety of "foreign bodies"—penises, babies, tampons—and these intrusions have made them more susceptible to problems. Transitional women are also a bit more likely to be taking antibiotics or other medications that may contribute to an infection.

Cervical/vaginal yeast infections are usually caused by Candida, a yeastlike fungus. There is always yeast in the vagina, but it is kept in check by the presence of vaginal bacteria, which maintain a normal, mildly acidic environment. When these bacteria are compromised—for example, if they are destroyed by a course of antibiotics—the yeast can proliferate unchecked in a more alkaline atmosphere and an infection occurs. Most of you have probably suffered the annoyance of a yeast infection by this time, but for those of you who've been lucky enough to escape, the symptoms include a thick white discharge, itching, burning, inflammation, redness, and pain.

To get rid of a yeast infection, derivatives of a family of medications called mycostatins work well, usually in the form of vaginal suppositories or cream. But yeast infections are tenacious. Spores can survive initial treatments, which is why it's often necessary to treat the infection more than once. I know some of my patients use home remedies such as yogurt, acidophilus cream, and vinegar, but in my experience, drugs are much more effective in eliminating the cause of the problem, at least for a longer period of time.

In the last couple of years, a whole crop of over-the-counter remedies for yeast infections has appeared on the market. Many of you have probably tried them. Unfortunately, though, they usually treat only one strain of yeast—*Candida albicans*—so if your problem is caused by another strain, they won't help. What's more, because women are overusing these products, we are seeing a growing number of infections caused by "more sophisticated" yeasts that are resistant to these over-the-counter drugs.

TRICHOMONIASIS AND VAGINOSIS. Trichomoniasis is another infection that can weaken your sex drive. It's caused by a protozoan called *Trichomonas vaginalis*. Symptoms include an unpleasant odor, a watery graying discharge, burning, and inflammation of the cervix and vaginal walls. Vaginosis, another common infection, also makes women less inclined to indulge in and enjoy sex. Caused by a bacterium, most commonly *Gardnerella vaginalis* (called G. vaginalis), it is accompanied by an irregular discharge and, sometimes, a burning sensation. You can contract both trichomoniasis and G. vaginalis from sexual contact.

The most effective way to treat trichomoniasis and

vaginosis is by taking a drug called metronidazole—you may know it by the brand name Flagyl. Both you and your sexual partner must be treated to bring about a lasting cure.

SEXUALLY TRANSMITTED DISEASES (STDs). STDs can compromise your health and interfere with your sex life. The following is a rundown of those you should know about.

- *Viral* STDs. Viral STDs are tricky because they cannot be cured with antibiotics and can only be treated symptomatically. They include:

HIV. The most deadly of all the sexually transmitted viruses is the human immunodeficiency virus (HIV), which causes acquired immune deficiency syndrome (AIDS). AIDS allows the body's immune system to become so severely impaired that it cannot fend off infection and disease. Because there's no cure for AIDS, "safe sex" can save your life; using a latex condom whenever you have intercourse is essential. Of course, the best way to prevent sexual transmission of HIV is abstinence.

HSV. Although not fatal, genital herpes simplex virus (HSV) is nonetheless distressing. HSV causes a raised pustule in the vagina that can be extremely painful when it is in its exacerbated state. (The pustule comes and goes; when it's present, it is in its "exacerbated" state.) This pustule can also occur in the cervix, but in that location it causes no pain, so you may never know you have it. There's no cure for HSV, either. Avoid transmission by not having sex when the pustule is present and/or by always using a condom.

HPV. Another STD is human papilloma virus (HPV), which causes a wartlike growth in the genital or pelvic area or cervix. Two types of HPV warts have been shown to be precancerous, but 90 percent of all HPV warts are benign. Still, if left alone they can grow so large—I've seen some as big as two inches in diameter—they can hinder sexual intercourse. They can also itch, hurt, and cause embarrassment.

Again, there's no cure for HPV. You can avoid transmission either by abstinence or use of a condom. Mild growths will often disappear on their own. If a growth becomes fairly sizable, your doctor will probably recommend removal, either by chemicals that "burn" it off or by cautery, surgery, or laser. Unfortunately, the warts often return in the same or in a nearby area.

• *Bacterial* STDs. The other major group of STDs around today is caused by bacteria. They are generally treatable *if* they are diagnosed.

GONORRHEA AND SYPHILIS. Don't get lulled into believing that gonorrhea and syphilis aren't a problem today. Not only do both exist, but in some places, they're on the rise. One of the reasons is that people in the early stages of these diseases show no symptoms, which makes it impossible for you to tell if your partner has either disease. Fortunately, though, both gonorrhea and syphilis can be treated with high doses of antibiotics. If you suspect you've been exposed, see your doctor immediately.

CHLAMYDIA AND MYCOPLASMOSIS. Chlamydia is a small bacteriumlike organism that usually appears with gonorrhea. Since we often find it in infertile women, doctors believe that chlamydia may damage the fallopian tubes and cause infertility.

Mycoplasma is a small bacterium that causes cervical and vaginal infections called mycoplasmosis. Research reveals that it may act like chlamydia in that it causes a vaginal discharge and also may be found in the fallopian tubes. Both chlamydia and mycoplasma can lead to *dyspareunia*, painful sexual intercourse.

Once detected through cervical DNA culture tests (cultures can be taken during an office visit), both chlamydia and mycoplasma can be cured by a full course of antibiotics, followed by four to six weeks of abstinence. Once again, using a condom or refraining from sex are the only methods of prevention.

It isn't easy to tell if your partner has an STD. Unless you happen to notice some sort of lesion or pustule, an acnelike blemish on your partner's penis or scrotum, or an unusual discharge from his penis—typical male symptoms of an acute STD—you (and he) may be totally unaware that he's infected. Another possibility: if you're not his only sexual partner, he may have become infected so recently that symptoms have not yet developed. However, he's still contagious. I urge you to ask any new lover if he has or ever has had an STD, as well as whether he's sexually active with others, even though I know you may not feel comfortable doing so.

In both women and men, the symptoms of an STD can seem so inconsequential that you don't even realize you're infected. It's important, therefore, to be alert for any of the following:

- *Unusual vaginal discharge on your underwear.*
- *Persistent moisture on the skin between your labia.*
- *Occasional mild pain in your pelvis.*
- *Burning or pain on urination.*
- *Or an unusual amount of discomfort caused by your doctor's routine pelvic exam.*

If you notice any of these, tell your doctor immediately. He or she can run blood tests and cultures that can detect the presence of an STD, and prescribe immediate treatment.

Even after treatment, tell your doctor if you see any unusual vaginal discharge, feel pain in your pelvic area, or experience burning or pain when you urinate. You'll want to be reevaluated to see whether or not you need more treatment. A sexually transmitted disease that is not successfully vanquished can lead to pelvic inflammatory disease (PID).

One more point: certain conditions, including yeast infections, trichomonas, and vaginalis, also can be transmitted sexually but are not classified as STDs. The reason is that these infections tend to stay localized in the genital area, whereas STDs such as syphilis or HIV can and often do affect the health of the entire body.

What seems like an explosion of sexually transmitted diseases has had both a positive and negative effect on the sex lives of transitional women. On the upside, it seems to have translated into more sexual fidelity. Infidelity, as we'll discuss in Chapter Twelve, is one of the reasons sex may nosedive in this time of your life, so loyalty is a definite plus. On the downside, however, the proliferation of STDs has put a damper on the sexual enthusiasm of many women, particularly those who are single. Some see celibacy as the only answer, but most transitional women aren't giving up sex altogether. Instead, they're becoming much more cautious when choosing a sexual partner.

Some people—particularly men who are trying to be persuasive—argue that being extremely cautious about sex is a defense mechanism that masks a fear of intimacy. The idea goes that since many women in their transitional years have already gone through at least one separation, divorce, or other such heartbreak, they are afraid to get involved.

STDs and AIDS have simply given them a valid and socially acceptable excuse to avoid more emotional pain.

This argument begs the question. Because AIDS is a sexually transmitted disease, and because AIDS is fatal, there *is* an inarguable connection between sex and death. Thus I believe that this sexual cautiousness stems more from good sense than from any emotional shortcoming. With all the STDs out there, you have good reason to take care. So I say "Stay wary" and take steps to keep yourself healthy.

Pelvic inflammatory disease (PID).

An infection or inflammation of the pelvic organs often caused by sexually transmitted diseases, PID may cause decreased sexual enjoyment. Symptoms range from a chronic, mild bellyache to severe pain in your pelvis or abdomen. You may even suffer from nausea, tiredness, lower back pain, foul-smelling vaginal discharge, irregular periods, and spotting. (For more on PID, see Chapter Ten.) Even after treatment with antibiotics, vaginal intercourse isn't recommended for at least six weeks to help insure that infection does not recur.

Vaginismus (vaginal spasms).

A perplexing and frustrating problem, vaginismus is characterized by painful spasms of the vagina brought about by involuntary, spasmodic contractions of the muscle that extends from the pubic bone to the coccyx (called the pubococcygeus) and related muscles surrounding the vaginal opening. Since the slightest touch can set off these spasms, sufferers cannot (nor do they desire to) have sexual intercourse. Among the causes of vaginismus are vaginal trauma (perhaps during childbirth or rape), ulcerations, and insufficient lubrication. It may also be triggered by a psychological aversion to intercourse.

The most effective treatment for vaginismus is two-pronged: psychological counseling for emotional causes and medical treatment for physical problems. The most popular medical remedy uses well-lubricated vaginal dilators of progressively larger sizes to enlarge the vagina. Often, muscle relaxants or nonsteroidal antiinflammatory drugs such as Advil or Motrin are used in conjunction with dilation treatment for added relief.

Gynecological Surgeries

The aftereffects of certain gynecological surgeries can also make you lose your desire for sex. If both of your ovaries are removed, estrogen levels plunge and you go into instant menopause. This can cause many of the other symptoms of estrogen deprivation we've discussed in earlier chapters, as well as a dry vagina, making intercourse unpleasant and unappealing.

Hysterectomy, too, may cause your sexual appetite to dull, although experts don't agree on why. Early research by Masters and Johnson suggested that during orgasm, the uterus elevates and then returns to its normal position. This has led some researchers to reason that if you don't have a uterus, you can't have an orgasm. These days, however, many sexologists dispute this idea. They say that a uterus is really not vital to sexual pleasure.

What most of us do agree on is that there's often some emotional distress following hysterectomy and that the surgery can affect a woman's sexual self-esteem. Some women say they feel less attractive and desirable, less "like a woman," after having this surgery. Some men fuel these feelings of inadequacy by treating their mates differently—less like an interesting and interested sex partner—not just during the healing period but for months, even years, afterward.

Hysterectomy is not the only procedure that can dramatically affect sexual feelings; mastectomy can also. Clearly, any cancer diagnosis can throw you into such an emotional maelstrom that having sex is the last thing on your mind. Radiation and chemotherapy can make you so debilitated that you just don't have the energy or enthusiasm for sex. But on top of all that, the loss of one or both breasts—in our society, the focal points of a woman's attractiveness—can severely damage a woman's entire self-image. Many mastectomy patients feel less sexy and attractive, particularly if they don't have the support and reassurance of a loving, understanding partner.

Surgery for cervical cancer may also trigger difficulties with heterosexual intercourse because it may lead to hysterectomy, often with actual shortening of the vagina. Thus, the penis may not be able to penetrate as deeply, particularly in the "missionary position." Unless you feel comfortable trying some other positions—such as side or rear entry—you may find yourself in a sexual slump.

What I want you to understand, however, is that you *can* enjoy satisfying sex after most surgeries. You should steer clear of sex for about six weeks immediately following surgery to give your body time to heal. After vaginal or cervical surgery, it's best to use a mild lipid lubricant such as K-Y Jelly for about a week or so once your sex life resumes. But after that you can and should feel free to enjoy!

Certain situations are somewhat more complicated. If the surgery caused any loss of ovarian activity, your body will suffer a loss of estrogen, with its accompanying vaginal dryness and atrophy. As I've already discussed, this problem can be remedied with estrogen replacement therapy to restore your hormone levels and/or lubrication.

Dealing with the emotional aftermath of gynecological surgery, however, can sometimes be more difficult. You may need to work on many sensitive and complex issues, such as restoring self-esteem, redefining a positive body image, and learning to communicate better with your mate—issues that can't be dealt with by a quick trip to your doctor's office or the drugstore. Working with a private mental health professional can help tremendously; so can joining a support group. Try to be patient. It takes time and commitment to work through the emotional hurdles gynecological surgery can create.

Chronic Illness

When you come down with the flu, complete with headache, fever, sneezing, watery eyes, sore throat, and stomach queasiness, the last thing in the world you want to do is have sex. Desire, however, usually returns when you feel better.

If you're chronically ill, you may seldom, or never, reach that feel-better stage, causing you to lose interest in sex at this time in your life. If your illness is well managed, however, sex may again seem appealing.

If you have mitral valve prolapse—a common, harmless condition in which the mitral valve in the heart sits lower than it should and doesn't close properly after each beat, leading to some minor irregularity in blood flow—you may suffer a drop in libido. The reason is not only that you may be more tired, but also that if you experience any palpitations, arrhythmias (irregular heartbeats), or, occasionally, even chest pain, you may shy away from sex for fear that the extra exertion may overtax your heart.

In most cases of chronic illness, including mitral valve prolapse, there's no medical reason why you should not have and enjoy good sex. Of course, you'll need to take the best possible care of yourself, following the wellness plan your doctor and good common sense prescribe. If a particular problem is getting in the way of good sex, you need to find the best way to remedy it. If you're too tired, for instance, taking vitamins, getting more exercise, and eating a diet high in carbohydrates and low in fat might help.

Equally important is to *believe* that you can still have great sex. It might help to keep in mind that sex may actually be *good* for you. It can provide a wonderful outlet for the tension and anxiety having a chronic ailment can cause. Sex also can offer you the comfort of touch, help you to feel more attractive and good about yourself, and even provide a healthful cardiovascular workout.

Endometriosis

Your sexual desire and enjoyment also can slip if you suffer from the persistent pelvic pain that can (but does not always) accompany endometriosis. With endometriosis—which can only be confirmed by laparoscopy—some of the tissue that normally lines the endometrium starts to grow in other parts of the body. I've seen endometriosis affect the outside of the uterus as well as the bladder, pelvic area, fallopian tubes, and ovaries. Endometriosis can cause not only pain but also excessive bleeding during menstruation.

Though it can't be cured, endometriosis is treatable. The simplest approach is usually birth control pills. If they don't bring relief, your doctor will probably try you on such anti-estrogens as danazol and tamoxifen. GnRH agonists such as Lupron and Synerol can also be effective.

If none of these methods work, surgery may. Growths are removed through laparoscopy with laser, cautery, and/or microsurgery. Occasionally, severe endometriosis may require a hysterectomy. Endometriomas, endometriosis within the ovary, require partial ovarian surgery or removal of the entire ovary.

Endometriosis is stubborn. If you stop taking your medications, it may recur. Sometimes it persists even after radical surgery. On the other hand, many transitional women find that as their estrogen decreases, their endometriosis improves. In fact, endometriosis usually disappears with the onset of menopause.

The Effect of Medications

Sometimes the medications you take to remedy certain ailments can actually create or at least exacerbate problems in your sex life. If you're taking propranolol or reserpine to combat high blood pressure, for instance, you can suffer a loss of libido. Some antidepressants, such as Tofranil, have been known to have the same effect, as have anti-anxiety drugs, including the old standard Valium. If you're on the Pill or are undergoing progesterone therapy, the progestins you're getting can also weaken your sexual desire.

If you're experiencing trouble having an orgasm, drugs could also be to blame. Amphetamines, found in some diet pills, and certain drugs prescribed for severe depression, including Nardil, Parnate, and Tofranil, can reduce your ability to have an orgasm.

When the Problem Is Emotional

If you're not as interested in sex as you used to be or shy away from intimacy even with a partner you love, and there doesn't seem to be any physical explanation, your problem may be emotional—or, as we say in the trade, psychosexual. Among transitional women, any of the following typically cause the libido to sag:

Infertility.

Reaching a point in your life when pregnancy is no longer easy, recommended, or, in some cases, even feasible can be an enormous blow to your sexual identity. The myth that a *real* woman is able to become pregnant—and that a *real* man will be able to impregnate her—puts enormous pressure on a heterosexual couple to conceive a child. If they don't succeed immediately, it can cause the self-esteem of both partners to plunge.

As a woman, you may feel less feminine and more unsure of yourself sexually if you are experiencing problems with infertility. You may also become more inhibited about expressing and enjoying yourself in the bedroom. Your male partner often feels equally inadequate and as a result may withdraw emotionally. Both reactions create distance at a time when closeness and communication are vital.

What's more, trying to conceive a child with the sex-by-the-clock scheduling that's often necessary in the transitional years isn't easy. It can take the romance and delight out of any sexual encounter, quickly turning it into a chore rather than a pleasure.

Miscarriage.

The risk of miscarriage escalates during the transitional years. Repeating miscarriages can be emotionally devastating. Understandably, many women are shaken by their inability to carry a child to term and by what they experience as the death of their baby. Many also become anxious about getting pregnant again and running the risk of losing yet another child. No wonder such repeated emotional trauma takes the joy out of heterosexual sex—intimacy becomes inextricably linked with failure and grief.

Infidelity.

In my practice, I hear more about infidelity from patients in their transitional years than I do from any other age group. Some women tell me their partners are cheating on them; some tell me they're afraid they may be pregnant—and their husband has had a vasectomy! Perhaps an affair relieves the boredom that may beset a long-term marriage. Maybe it's a way to express anger with a spouse, or a misguided attempt to boost sagging self-esteem and reaffirm attractiveness by drawing the attentions of another sexual partner.

Infidelity is caused by several stressors that mesh in the transitional years. Women at this stage of life may find they've hit the glass ceiling, so they may feel frustrated and unappreciated at work. They may have a child who is readying to leave the nest, which may make them feel less needed and valuable, or maybe they're trying to become pregnant and having a tough time of it, which can threaten their sense of womanliness and self-esteem.

Additionally, most transitional women have reached a stage of life where they're beginning to take stock of themselves. Part of that stock-taking involves reevaluating the quality of their intimate relationships both in and out of bed. Transitional women say to themselves, "Am I as happy as I could be? Am I as sexually satisfied as I could be? Am I as emotionally fulfilled as I could be? Does my partner care about my needs? Does my companion show me the concern and consideration I feel I deserve?"

If the answer to any one of these questions is no, they may turn to someone outside of their central relationship to find the satisfaction they are seeking and reaffirm that they are sexy, attractive, and worthwhile. Meanwhile, their mates may be doing the same thing. So what we often see is a breakdown of trust between partners in the transitional years that powerfully affects their sexual lives in a negative way.

Stress.

Forty-year-old Karen has a problem typical of women in their transitional years—an overwhelming number of demands and responsibilities that have led to physical and emotional exhaustion. "I'm incredibly busy," says Karen. "I have a seven-year-old and a toddler to take care of and a demanding career in sales which involves very long hours. Recently, my father died, and my mother, who is not well, moved in with us. By the time I get home, take care of the family, eat dinner, tidy up, and prepare for the next day, I'm half dead. When I get into bed, the last thing I want to think about, much less have, is sex."

In a slightly different way, emotional stress is also taking its toll on Diane, a divorced, forty-four year old. "I work all day and while I don't have any kids or a husband to worry about when I get home, I just don't have the energy to go out socializing. Plus, between AIDS and the lack of available men out there, even if I had the energy, I don't see much opportunity. You want to know about my sex life? Let's put it this way: The last time I had sex Carter was president! I'm kidding, but it has been a while. You know, it's more the intimacy and the closeness I miss than the sex itself. My sex drive seems to have cooled. You know the phrase 'Use it or lose it'? Well, I think I'm losing it!"

Boredom.

Couples who've been together for a while may find themselves tired of the same old sex, done in the same old way. It's one of the pitfalls of knowing each other very well. The trick is to recognize this problem and take action to break out of your tiresome routine.

Embarrassment.

Even in these days of Madonna, steamy TV love scenes, and condoms in the classrooms, men and women are often embarrassed to talk about their sexual needs and preferences. Many women worry that if they bare their souls along with their bodies, their partner may think they're deviant or "too experienced," as one patient confided. So asking for what they want in bed becomes taboo.

Worry over sexual performance.

There's a scene in Woody Allen's movie *Manhattan* that I really like. Woody's character is at a chic cocktail party and the subject turns to orgasm. As the guests trade quips, one young, somewhat empty-headed woman announces, "I had an orgasm once. But my doctor said it was the wrong kind."

Funny as that line is, it holds a sad truth. Many of my patients confide anxiously that they're not sure they've ever had an orgasm, or worry that the orgasms they do have aren't intense enough. I'm not sure why so many women feel this way. Maybe well-meaning sexologists writing in popular magazines and appearing on talk shows have just placed too much emphasis on the almighty orgasm. Whatever the reason, the result is this: many women have become so uptight about whether or not a sexual encounter will lead to an orgasm that they can't allow themselves to simply relax and enjoy the intimacy.

Strategies to Spice Up Your Sex Life

When psychosexual problems are behind the loss of your sexual zest, there's no quick and easy cure. Coping successfully with any of the issues I've just described is mostly a matter of learning to relax and communicate more openly with your partner. In some cases, you may also need a sex education refresher course—new positions and sexual techniques—to rev you up. But remember: as a transitional woman, you have the capacity to enjoy the best sex you ever had. Here are a few suggestions that can help you tap that potential.

Take a break!

Living a life so crammed full of demands and responsibilities can throw perspective and priorities out of sync. Take some time out. Stop trying to conceive for a month or two. Go on a vacation, even if it's only a long weekend at a bed and breakfast. If you've been with your partner for a while, taking some time off to remember why you two got together in the first place can be an important first step in reestablishing communication and caring.

Simplify your life.

Trying to do too much takes its toll on your emotional energy and your sexual desires. Vacations and time-outs are terrific, but at some point the day-to-day grind begins again. To help insure that you won't fall into the same traps, see if there's a way to simplify your life by eliminating some of your less important commitments and responsibilities. So what if the house isn't as tidy as you'd like? Do you have to stay late at the office every night? Can you drop out of that social committee for a while? The goal here: get rid of all excess responsibilities so that you can get back to what matters again.

Learn to relax.

This isn't the first time you've heard me say this and it won't be the last. Learning how to relax and unwind often has a remarkable effect: it makes you feel more sexy. Deep breathing, meditation, exercise, and yoga are all wonderful relaxation techniques. Try any of them for fifteen minutes twice a day for six weeks—it takes six weeks to break a bad habit and just as long to create a good one—and see if it doesn't make you feel more desirous and desirable.

Make time for sex.

If you don't have sex for long periods of time, you begin to desire it less. So if you have a mate and you've both been too busy to find room for sex in your life, make some. Schedule a night or afternoon together, write it down in your appointment book if necessary, but as the commercial says, "Just do it." You'll be surprised to find how one such "date" leads to another.

If you don't have a partner, manual masturbation is satisfying. Another option: use a mechanical device such as a vibrator; just be careful not to cause any physical damage or to inflict pain.

Learn to express your needs.

Getting the most from your sexual encounters means learning how to ask your partner to do what pleases you, whether it's tickling your toes with a feather or kissing that erogenous spot on your neck. If you're too embarrassed and uncomfortable to communicate your needs, no one will ever know what they are.

If sex embarrasses you, try desensitizing yourself by renting some "blue" movies to watch at home, or listening to sexually explicit audio tapes over and over again. Joining a support group (choose it carefully) can also help; hearing others talk about sexual intimacies eventually helps you to become more comfortable saying the words yourself. After a while, you'll be able to bring your newfound ease into the bedroom. Once you start telling your partner how to fulfill your needs and desires, chances are you'll get an enthusiastic response.

Quit worrying about orgasm.

Let's set the record straight. There's nothing mysterious about an orgasm. It simply consists of three responses:

1. Some reaction of the sympathetic nervous system (the muscles and nerves you don't consciously control)—such as

contractions of smooth muscles in your pelvis and breasts—and other physiological changes such as sweating.

2. An increase of tension, arousal, and emotions that build to a peak.

3. A release of those feelings and a gradual return to normal.

Pretty general, don't you think? And that's precisely the point: *There's no defined entity that is the perfect orgasm.* Since every individual is different, orgasmic response varies greatly from person to person. What is satisfactory for you may not be for someone else; some women are happy at one level, others at another.

I think phrases like "achieving orgasm" set women (and men) on the wrong course. All you want to do is reach a point of emotional and physical tension—then release—that *feels* good. To allow yourself to feel good, of course, it's important to have sex in a comfortable setting. You probably won't be at ease in that squeaky sofa bed at your in-laws'. Once you find a place that's right for you—whether a heart-shaped bed in the Poconos or your own living room couch—it becomes much easier to just enjoy the moment without trying to *achieve* anything. If you simply concentrate on making you and your partner feel good, your sexual satisfaction will increase tenfold.

Experiment.

If your sexual relationship is boring and unimaginative, try adding some zip by experimenting with new positions or techniques. There are many excellent sex manuals in print; peruse them at your local bookstore and choose one that feels right to you. Certain videos, too, offer sexual pointers.

Consult a sexual therapist.

He or she can help you and your mate improve your lovemaking through such techniques as *nongenital sensate focus*, which simply means using a variety of methods to arouse yourself and your partner that don't directly involve the genitals. Nongenital sensate focus includes massage, applying sensual oils and lotions to each other's bodies, washing each other's hair—whatever feels really good but does not directly stimulate your sexual organs. This technique will not only feel wonderful but will help you lose some of your inhibitions and thereby deepen your sexual pleasure. By the way, sex therapists report pretty good success with this kind of therapy; they assert that as many as 75 to 80 percent of those instructed in nongenital sensate focus say it heightened their sexual enjoyment.

Tisha, thirty-nine, and Rob, forty-eight, are a case in point. They were floundering with their sex life for over a year. After a short session with a sex therapist, during which several suggestions were offered, they took a long weekend at a bed and breakfast at the seashore and dedicated their time to sex. They brought along a bottle of a sweet-smelling oil and gave each other long, sensual massages. Later on, they experimented with some new positions the therapist had recommended and found they excited them enormously.

"Suddenly," Tisha told me about a year later, "all those months of bad sex or no sex just melted away. We really felt renewed. And now whenever our sex drive gets stuck in low gear, we take some scented candles, a bottle of that wonderful oil, hop in the car, and head for some little B&B to rediscover ourselves."

Seek psychological counseling.

Sometimes airing your problems under the guidance of a trained psychotherapist is an excellent way to open up lines of communication between you and your mate. Ask your doctor for the name of a qualified professional—a psychologist, psychiatrist, social worker, or marriage counselor—who could work with you as a couple.

Men's Sexual Problems

While this book spotlights transitional women and not transitional men (if there is such a thing), it's hard to talk about sexuality without focusing, albeit briefly, on the opposite sex. After all, in a heterosexual relationship, both the woman *and* the man play a part.

A man's sexual ability typically peaks in early adulthood. By the time he's reached his mid to late thirties and beyond—the years when he's most likely to have a relationship with a transitional woman—he may be experiencing a number of changes in his sexual capabilities that affect *your* sexual responsiveness and enjoyment as his partner.

The most benign and commonplace of these changes lies in his ability to get, maintain, and, after orgasm, quickly regain an erection. In the young man, all stages of the sexual act—excitement, plateau, orgasm, and resolution—are quite short. As he moves into his late thirties, forties, and fifties, these stages become more prolonged, but his refractory period—that is, the time it takes for his erection to return after orgasm—changes most of all. Although there is great individual variation, in general a more mature male will take a good deal longer to regain his erection than the few moments it took him when he was in his teens and early twenties.

Most of these changes are the normal result of growing older. But some men experience certain sexual shifts—dysfunctions, actually—that can really hurt a couple's sex life. These are the most common:

Erection loss.

Some men can get an erection but have trouble keeping it; others lose their ability to get any erection at all.

Premature ejaculation.

A man with this problem ejaculates almost immediately after becoming sexually aroused, long before his partner or, in some cases, the couple have orgasm.

Sexual dysphoria.

Some men can get turned on only by playing out a fantasy. When that fantasy is not desired by both partners—for example, handcuffing or whipping a partner during sex—the man is said to be suffering from a sexual dysphoria.

Fantasy loss.

In order for a man to get an erection, he usually needs to fantasize. (This doesn't mean he's fantasizing about someone else; he is often thinking only about you.) When he loses the ability to fantasize, it becomes more difficult if not impossible for him to become erect.

Obviously, some of these problems make the ability to engage in certain sexual acts, particularly intercourse, physically difficult. All can trigger emotional distress. A man who is having problems getting an erection may become so tense and anxious before going to bed with his partner that he will simply avoid the situation and shun sex altogether.

I've always found most transitional women to be quite sensitive to their partner's sexual difficulties and the feelings of inadequacy they may generate in him. Prolonged problems, however, may cause even the most understanding woman to get angry and frustrated at her mate for not being able to satisfy her sexual needs. Some women may get offended, mistakenly interpreting their partner's problems as a sign that he's losing interest in them. In turn, that makes them feel less attractive; they may even start blaming themselves for their partner's difficulties. I've heard many of my patients say, "If only I were more attractive [or thinner, younger, more voluptuous—the list goes on and on], he would not have these problems." Such feelings often begin a downward spiral into less frequent and less pleasurable sex—and an unhappy interpersonal relationship.

Help for Men

Occasionally, male sexual dysfunction stems from a health problem such as a urinary tract infection, a prostate ailment, or a decrease in the level of the male hormone testosterone. Sometimes medications, including blood pressure medications, painkillers, steroids, antihistamines, or antibiotics, are the culprits. Once uncovered, these problems can be managed successfully.

When the trouble stems from an emotional problem, such as depression or anxiety, treatment isn't that simple. Usually some form of psychological counseling is the most effective route, either individually or in couple therapy. Sometimes, psychotherapy works best in conjunction with some kind of drug treatment, such as taking antidepressants or anti-anxiety medications, although special care must be taken since some of these drugs can weaken sexual desire.

Sex therapy with a trained sexologist may help, too. Basically, sex therapy involves raising body awareness and arousal. Sometimes, the therapist will encourage patients to view X-rated videotapes or read sexually explicit magazines. Other techniques involve music or verbal stimulation. Masturbation is usually recommended; there is evidence that successful masturbation is associated with sexual success with a partner.

For premature ejaculation, instruction in nongenital sensate focus is often helpful. So is the stop-start technique, in which the man is stimulated until just prior to ejaculation, when the stimulation is stopped. Once he relaxes, stimulation begins again. The process is repeated until he eventually becomes better at controlling when he ejaculates. Another good tactic is learning various ways to be sexually intimate, including oral sex and different positions for intercourse.

Men who can't get or maintain an erection may do well with *genital sensate focus*, a fancy term for learning various techniques for stimulating the genitals either orally or manually. This stimulation does seem to be effective in helping a man control his ability to stay erect.

Most times, revitalizing your sexual self demands a multifaceted approach. First, you need to discover if there's any physical or medical basis for your problems. But since sex takes place 95 percent between the ears, it's important to consider any emotional or psychological issues that may be relevant, too. Once you discover the source of the difficulty and work to remedy it, the payoff is big: a rich and zestful sexual life you'll enjoy for more years than you ever thought possible.

8

Managing Estrogen- and Age-Related Medical Conditions

- Fibrocystic Breast Disease (FCD)
- Osteoporosis: Are Your Bones in Trouble?
- Neurogenic Aging Symptoms (NAS)
- A Recommendation to Take Action

We've talked a lot about estrogen's role in keeping your reproductive system in good shape. The effects of this powerful hormone, however, reach well beyond your ovaries and uterus. Estrogen affects the health of your breasts, bones, brain, and nervous system as well. Each is strongly influenced by estrogen, so any change in the amount or activity level of this hormone can trigger some troublesome conditions.

Age, too, plays a role. As you get older and enter the transitional years, estrogen levels begin to fluctuate significantly, thus placing transitional women at special risk for certain medical conditions. Specifically, three key problems—fibrocystic breast disease, osteoporosis, and neurogenic aging symptoms—either appear or intensify during this time of your life, depending upon how your body responds to its changing estrogen levels.

While not directly life-threatening, any of these conditions can—and often do—reduce the quality of a woman's life. But it's not a given. Each problem can be managed, thanks to new techniques and treatments. Sometimes the hardest part is identifying the problem in the first place. Symptoms can be so subtle that accurate diagnosis is difficult—which is why the more you know about each of these conditions, the better off you'll be.

Fibrocystic Breast Disease (FCD)

One of the most common problems of the transitional years is an increase in fibrocystic disease, a breast complaint that is affected by both aging and fluctuating estrogen levels. The older you get and the further you move from your peak reproductive years, the greater your risk. Further, decreasing levels of estrogen can intensify FCD—which is why it's estimated that 50 percent of all transitional women suffer from this problem.

Actually, fibrocystic disease isn't a disease at all. It's simply a breast condition marked by a particular set of physiological changes.

The breasts of a woman with normal menstrual cycles have a cycle all their own. Prior to ovulation, increasing estrogen levels cause the mammary ducts to widen. After ovulation, when both estrogen and progesterone are available, there is a marked increase in both the size and number of cells within the breast ducts, and the amount of secretions flowing within them. These changes are most apparent just before your period, when estrogen and progesterone levels are high. Once the hormone levels fall, the breasts return to their smaller size and state within twenty-four hours.

Many women have such remarkable breast activity during their cycle that over time the ducts become overextended or damaged and can't return to normal. The connective tissue surrounding the ducts tries to correct this damage by forming a network of fiberlike tissues (*fibrosis*) around the ducts.

The problem also occurs as the body's estrogen levels begin to drop during the transitional years. When estrogen levels decrease to the point where they fail to bring about ovulation, and, therefore, progesterone is not produced—a situation that occurs more frequently after age thirty-five—the estrogen that does exist is unopposed by progesterone. This unchecked estrogen results in additional irregular growth of fibrous tissue.

What's more, the secretions in the damaged breast ducts often become trapped, forming small to large fluid-filled lumps called breasts cysts. When there are both fibrosis and cystic changes, you have FCD.

Although FCD isn't life-threatening, symptoms can be troublesome enough to prompt some sufferers to seek treatment. FCD can cause breast pain and soreness, usually from ovulation to menstruation, when the bumpy and enlarged breasts that mark FCD are at their fullest. (If you don't ovulate, pain could occur at any time in your cycle, depending upon when estrogen levels surpass a certain threshold. But that threshold varies enormously from person to person.)

FCD can also make mammography less efficient, because its benign lumps or cysts can obscure malignancies that may lie behind them. To give yourself the best chance for an accurate mammogram, never have one just before, during, or immediately following your period. You'll get the most reliable readings from about three days after your period until the middle of your cycle.

As I've already explained, FCD is more likely to occur—or, if you've had it before, to become more prominent—during the transitional years. However, there's good news in store. Once estrogen drops off completely in menopause and there is no activity in the breast tissue, the symptoms of FCD disappear. Hormone therapy, however, can cause some mild FCD symptoms to occur.

More encouraging data: although we used to believe that women with FCD were at greater risk for breast cancer, recent research has now thrown that conclusion into doubt. Women with the benign breast lumps characteristic of FCD seem to be at no greater risk for breast cancer than women without this condition.

Is it cancer?

How can you tell if a breast lump is merely a symptom of FCD and not cancer?

Answer: you can't. But until you receive confirmation from your doctor, here are some facts that may give you peace of mind.

1. The bumps that mark FCD usually shrink in size or seem to disappear completely after your period. Malignancies rarely shrink and never disappear.

2. FCD lumps tend to be very sore. Most malignancies are not.

3. When you touch a benign lump, it's hard to tell precisely where it begins and ends; with malignancies you feel definite boundaries.

4. If you discover lumps in both breasts, it's less likely to be cancer than if you find a lump in one.

Keep in mind, however, that no one, not even the most highly qualified physician, can tell for certain if a lump is malignant simply by feeling it. To rule out any suspicions of cancer, your doctor will probably want you to have a few tests—first, a mammogram; then, if necessary, an ultrasound, which can usually help determine if the lump is filled with water. If a solid tumor is suspected, you may undergo a surgical biopsy in which all of a small lump, or part of a large one, is removed and sent to a lab for analysis. Sometimes, if your doctor can't actually feel the lump, he or she will do an X-ray assisted biopsy. The X-ray helps to locate the problem, and the minimal dosage of radiation you get from such X-rays is far outweighed by the potential of detecting a malignancy at an early stage.

Another possibility is a needle biopsy. In this procedure, your doctor inserts a needle into the lump and removes some of the tissue by suction. The tissue is then sent to a lab for analysis. This procedure is simpler and less traumatic than a surgical biopsy, but it has 90 to 95 percent accuracy as opposed to 100 percent for surgery. Whatever approach you and your doctor choose, however, you should have the results of the biopsy within forty-eight to seventy-two hours.

Treating fibrocystic breast disease.

Not every women with FCD needs or wants treatment. Often, symptoms are so mild—occasional breast soreness or tenderness a few days each month—that you simply choose to live with them. That's fine. FCD does *not* require treatment. If you find the symptoms more bothersome, however, you have a few treatment options available.

THE CAFFEINE CONNECTION. While there are no documented studies that confirm a link between caffeine and FCD, abundant anecdotal evidence indicates that reducing caffeine intake helps relieve the problems associated with FCD. Many of my patients tell me that when they cut back on caffeine—reducing or completely eliminating coffee, colas, and chocolate from their diet—their symptoms abated pretty dramatically. Maria, a thirty-eight-year-old hairdresser, is a perfect example.

While examining her breasts one month, Maria felt a large lump about the size of a small plum. She'd known for years that she had FCD, but this lump was so large it really scared her. So she made an immediate appointment.

An ultrasound revealed a large mass in the area where she'd felt the lump. I was certain from the ultrasound that the lump contained fluid, so I inserted a fine needle into the mass and aspirated (removed) the fluid. This caused the lump to disappear, and Maria was greatly relieved. Her lump had been nothing more than a benign cyst.

After this scare, Maria, a coffee drinker and chocoholic, eliminated caffeine from her diet. She switched to decaf and cut out chocolate. Nine months later, not only hasn't her cyst returned, but her breasts are considerably less lumpy and tender than before.

VITAMINS. Making sure you have adequate vitamins in your diet also seems to relieve FCD. Specifically, many women find taking daily doses of vitamins C (500 milligrams), E (400 IU), A (5,000 IU), and B_6 (2.0 milligrams) brings welcome relief.

MEDICATIONS. To alleviate pain, you can also try small doses of anti-prostaglandins, such as ibuprofen-based Advil, Nuprin, Motrin, or, if your doctor prescribes it, 275 milligrams of naproxin-based Anaprox.

HORMONE TREATMENTS. Since lumps and cysts are produced by an excess of estrogen at a certain point in your cycle, anti-estrogens such as danazol (brand name Danocrine), tamoxifen citrate (brand name Nolvadex), and gestrinone can soothe severe "mastodynia," extremely painful breasts. Very low doses are given in order to reduce the likelihood of such unpleasant side effects as hot flashes or the growth of hair on your face or other undesirable places. I prefer to give anti-estrogens for only two to three months (on a daily basis). Taking anti-estrogens over a longer period of time could reduce too drastically transitional women's already declining estrogen levels. Another drawback to anti-estrogens: they're expensive.

If your FCD discomfort is limited to a few days before your period or just after ovulation, it may be due to inadequate progesterone. Small doses of Provera—2.5 milligrams taken once or twice a day whenever you feel discomfort in your breasts—may help reduce or even eliminate your symptoms.

You may have heard or read about some doctors treating FCD with thyroid hormone and cortisone. But I don't recommend this approach for the simple reason that it just doesn't seem to work.

IODINE THERAPY. Research conducted by Dr. William Ghent, professor of surgery at Queens University in Kingston, Ontario, and me suggests that iodine may also work to relieve FCD. In about 80 to 90 percent of cases of severe breast pain, a special form of iodine taken orally reduced soreness and fibrocystic changes in the breast with minimal side effects. While iodine treatment is already being used to some extent in Canada, it's still in trial in the United States. But if all continues to go well, it may be offered here fairly soon.

According to the American Academy of Pathology, 80 percent of all North American women in their reproductive years have FCD, at least to some degree. And fully 35 to 45 percent of all women diagnosed with the problem need treatment. If you think you might be one of them, I urge you to talk with your doctor. As I've explained, much can be done to alleviate any suffering.

Osteoporosis: Are Your Bones in Trouble?

Undoubtedly, you have at least some idea of what osteoporosis is all about. Because women in the transitional years are at greater risk for this disease than their younger counterparts, you owe it to yourself to understand it in greater detail so you can lower your chances for future problems and make informed choices about treatment if and when you need to.

Osteoporosis literally means "porous bones." It's a condition characterized by a decrease in bone mass—a thinning of your bones—which makes you vulnerable to fractures, particularly of the vertebrae, hip, and pelvis. It also impedes motion of the long bones; that is, the bones in your arms and legs. In severe cases, doing something as simple as lifting a bag of groceries could cause you to break a bone in your arm or wrist.

Because osteoporosis often affects the spinal column, it can also cause nagging backaches and rounded shoulders. In fact, one of the recognizable hallmarks of severe osteoporosis—underscoring its prevalence among older women—is the "dowager's hump," caused by compressed fractures of the upper spine. (Men, too, can get osteoporosis, but it is rare and does not usually occur until they're over seventy.)

After age thirty-five, bone mass in women decreases by about 1 to 2 percent each year. If the amount of mass you started out with is substantial—if your calcium intake is adequate, and if your estrogen levels remain sufficiently high to help bones keep restoring themselves, at least to some extent—this gradual decline doesn't matter all that much. As estrogen decreases, however, so does your bones' ability to regenerate themselves. If your bone mass wasn't that great to begin with, your risk for osteoporosis soars. A cumulative loss of only 15 to 20 percent of bone mass is enough to cause deformities, such as a humped back or bowed legs.

Are you at risk?

Your risk for osteoporosis goes up if you have any of the following:

- *Family history of osteoporosis.*
- *Light skin.* Caucasian women are at greater risk than women of color.
- *Proximity to menopause.* The closer you are to menopause and the lower your estrogen levels, the higher your risk.
- *Low calcium intake.*
- *Liver or kidney disease.*

- *Many pregnancies.*
- *Sedentary, high-stress job.*
- *Lack of exercise.*

Some scientists believe that measuring your actual bone mass is a much better gauge than analyzing the above risk factors, which are associated with osteoporosis but do not guarantee that you'll have trouble. They believe it's possible to predict whether or not you'll get osteoporosis through a process called *densitometry*, or *absorptiometry*.

In densitometry, complex instruments are used to perform one of two painless procedures: single-photon absorptiometry, which measures the density of the bones in your forearm, wrist, and heel; and dual-photon absorptiometry, which assesses the condition of the bones in your hip and spine. These tests indicate how much of your bone mass has been lost already. From this information, doctors can estimate how much you're likely to lose in the future.

The jury is still out on how reliable these tests are. Right now, I don't believe that their accuracy justifies their expense, but some orthopedic surgeons and doctors at certain women's clinics are using them, so if you have reason to be worried about osteoporosis, these tests are available to you.

There is one reliable way to measure bone density: CAT (computerized axial tomography) scan. A CAT scan of the spine can lead to an accurate assessment of bone loss, but because of the radiation involved and the costliness of this procedure, this test is not used to measure a seemingly healthy woman's risk for osteoporosis.

What causes osteoporosis.

The key cause of bone loss is a calcium deficiency. Your bones consist of two types of cells: *osteoclasts*, which break down the bone, and *osteoblasts*, which make the bone grow. This breaking down and building up of bone occurs throughout your lifetime. In order for osteoblasts to form good bone, sufficient calcium needs to be present and usable.

When calcium enters the body, it is absorbed from your gastrointestinal tract into your bloodstream. Any excess is either excreted by the kidneys or deposited in the ends of the bone shafts, where it is saved in a kind of storage bin until your body needs it. The problem is that once you reach age thirty-five, you can no longer add to your calcium reserve, which means you have a limited amount of calcium present in your body. Each time you need some extra calcium—say, for example, to help repair damage caused by a simple fracture like a broken finger—you begin to deplete your reserves and place yourself at slightly greater risk for reduced bone mass.

Now here's where you can see estrogen's impact. Estrogen influences osteoblastic activity and helps maintain bone mass. When estrogen levels decrease, so does the ability of your osteoblasts to form new bone. Decreasing levels of estrogen also affect your body's ability to utilize vitamin D in the formation of new bone. Because estrogen also helps to activate vitamin D (through a chemical reaction, vitamin D is converted into vitamin D_3, which your body can then use to get your osteoblasts moving), decreasing amounts of estrogen have a doubly harmful effect on your body's ability to form bone.

Loss of calcium, weaker and less active osteoblasts, and lowered estrogen all combine to cause an imbalance in the bone. That gives osteoclasts the upper hand and causes your bones to have less mass and, therefore, to become weaker and more porous.

Another factor may make matters worse: studies suggest that progesterone aids in bone formation and that women who do not produce enough progesterone—either because they're not ovulating or because they have a shortened secretory phase in their menstrual cycle (therefore trimming the time period in which progesterone is available)—may also be at risk for osteoporosis. As you may remember from Chapter Three, lack of ovulation and a disturbed menstrual cycle are common problems for transitional women.

Other causes of decreased bone mass include:

- *An excess of protein in your diet.* The presence of protein in the bowel can hamper calcium absorption. You only need 44 grams of protein daily, which is the equivalent of about six ounces of meat.
- *The natural aging process.* Aging often makes the intestines less effective in absorbing calcium, and makes the kidneys filter out more calcium during urination.
- *Alcohol and tobacco use.* These substances interfere with calcium absorption. Marijuana use is also thought to be detrimental to bone production.
- *Drinking too much carbonated soda.* Avoid sodas containing phosphate, a chemical that acts against calcium in the bloodstream, reducing its efficiency in helping form new bone. To identify sodas containing phosphate, look for the words *phosphate* or *phosphoric acid* in the list of ingredients. If you can't resist drinking these sodas, keep your intake to no more than two cans per day.
- *Hyperthyroidism.* An overactive thyroid could cause calcium to pass through your intestines too rapidly, before it can be sufficiently absorbed. An abnormally functioning thyroid gland also secretes less *calcitonin*, a hormone that helps in calcium metabolism. This again hampers your body's ability to use calcium to build and strengthen bones.

Preventing osteoporosis.

Perhaps the scariest aspect of osteoporosis is that the loss of bone mass occurs silently, so that you may never know it's happening until the disease is fairly advanced. Osteoporosis is treatable, but not curable, so your best weapon against this secretive enemy is prevention—which is why it's so important to follow these guidelines:

- *Make sure your daily diet includes 800 milligrams of calcium.* Good sources of calcium are green leafy vegetables; dairy products such as low-fat or nonfat yogurt and skim milk, and low-fat cheese; and certain types of fish, such as sardines (with bones) and salmon. A cup of yogurt contains about 400 milligrams of calcium; a cup of milk, about 300 milligrams; a half cup of broccoli or kale equals about 175 milligrams of calcium; and three ounces of sardines (with bones), about 200 milligrams.
- *Make up for any deficiencies in your diet by taking calcium in the form of supplements,* plus vitamins D (5 milligrams) and C (60 milligrams), which encourage calcium absorption.
- *Exercise regularly.* Weight-bearing activities, such as aerobics, hiking, jogging, and walking, work to increase bone density because bones get bigger when they're forced to deal with added stress. Exercise also helps to increase circulation and get needed nutrients to your bones.

As I've stressed in earlier chapters, while you should exercise three to five times a week, don't overdo it. Excessive exercise can cause estrogen levels to drop, which can put you at greater risk for bone loss.

Treating osteoporosis.

Even if you develop osteoporosis, there are some effective ways to find relief.

- *Pain medications.* Women in mild pain can take aspirin, Advil, Motrin, Anaprox, or even, under a doctor's strict supervision, such mild narcotics as codeine.
- *Synthetic Salmon Calcitonin (SCT).* Recent research has revealed some encouraging data about synthetic salmon calcitonin, a chemical that has the same effect as natural calcitonin, a thyroid hormone found in salmon that aids in bone and calcium absorption. Apparently, SCT slows down bone loss by weakening osteoclasts, the cells that break down bone, and by strengthening the bone-building osteoblasts. What's more, biweekly injections of SCT may actually reduce bone pain resulting from osteoporosis. Beware, though: SCT treatments are very expensive.
- *Biphosphonates.* Another promising treatment—so new that it's still in the experimental stage—involves chemicals called biphosphonates. These drugs seem to build up osteoblasts while reducing osteoclasts. The big problem is that they have some dangerous side effects, including potential damage to the liver and kidneys. If scientists can figure out how to reduce or eliminate these harmful effects, biphosphonates may offer great hope to thousands of women.
- *Hormones.* Many patients have found relief through estrogen supplement therapy. Taking 0.3 milligrams of Premarin supplements their own estrogen supply enough to relieve many of the problems associated with osteoporosis. Usually, however, estrogen therapy works best in conjunction with other treatments.

Ilene is a case in point. She was thirty-eight years old when she went to see a colleague of mine, another gynecologist, complaining of hot flashes and pain in her pelvic bone. The pelvic pain was occurring more and more often, Ilene told him, and occasionally lasted for several days. First, the doctor prescribed estrogen supplement therapy for Ilene. Then, suspecting osteoporosis, he suggested a dual-photon absorption test, which confirmed his suspicion: evidence of bone mass loss that, if not halted as soon as possible, could lead to further difficulties down the road.

To treat the problem, Ilene was given calcium supplements and encouraged to go on a strict exercise regimen. One year later, another dual-photon absorption test showed substantial improvement; there was a marked increase in bone mass in the areas evaluated. Today, she no longer takes the supplements, but she still monitors her diet to make sure she's getting enough calcium and continues to exercise regularly.

Other hormone strategies that have worked include estrogen/progesterone cycling (in which you take estrogen alone for a few days, then add progesterone as well) and taking birth control pills. (For more details on these treatments, see Chapter Three.)

If you're into natural remedies, you might want to investigate plant estrogens. These "phyto-estrogens" appear to behave similarly to the body's natural estrogen and, therefore, seem to have comparable effects. As a physician, I can't offer you recommendations on specific dosages, but I can tell you that phyto-estrogens are found in such plants as elder, sarsaparilla, and licorice. You can brew them in water and drink them as tea. If you want to try phyto-estrogens, find a health care professional, such as a nutritionist skilled in natural treatments, to guide you. Just be sure to let your medical doctor know your intentions; that way he or she won't prescribe too many additional hormones and overload your system.

Neurogenic Aging Symptoms (NAS)

Many of my patients in their transitional years complain of headaches, memory problems, a change in their senses of smell and taste, and lowered stamina. In fact, I've heard these complaints so often that I've grouped them together under the term Neurogenic Aging Symptoms (NAS).

You won't find NAS mentioned in any medical text or professional journal. Neurogenic Aging Symptoms is a phrase I coined to refer to certain complaints that, while quite distinct from each other, are all related, at least to some degree, to changes in your brain and nervous system (thus the term *neurogenic*) as you grow older (thus the word *aging*). I've included NAS in this chapter because clinical and anecdotal evidence suggests a connection between lowered estrogen levels and the onset of these symptoms in transitional women.

The symptoms of NAS.

HEADACHES. Migraine headaches, which are usually vascular in nature—meaning they're caused by problems involving the blood vessels in your head—are *not* part of NAS. But your basic, garden-variety, stress-related, nonvascular head-pounders most certainly are. While no one knows for sure what causes these headaches, I am convinced they are related to changes in estrogen level. As estrogen begins to decrease in your transitional years, headaches may start to occur more frequently.

One explanation is that estrogen seems to get into your brain by means of certain substances called *catecholamine-estrogens*. (Catecholamines are the substances that chemically stimulate your nerves.) When there's a reduction of estrogen, certain catecholamines do not respond properly and thus do not stimulate your brain and nerve centers adequately. The theory is that certain brain waves are inhibited, triggering headaches as well as some memory loss.

Much of this information is speculative, however. More research needs to be conducted before we can truly understand estrogen's impact on the brain and nervous system. Even so, I believe that we already have enough data to support the idea that estrogen exerts some measure of influence.

SHORT-TERM MEMORY LOSS. You may have already noticed this problem, without realizing it is one that belongs to NAS. You make out a shopping list and forget to bring it to the grocery store; you go into a room for a specific reason, but as soon as you get there, forget why. You remember what you wore to your senior prom, but can't remember the name of the actress who starred in the movie you saw last night.

Short-term memory lapses are probably caused, at least in part, by an estrogen/brain interaction that is similar to the one that may cause NAS headaches. Animal studies conducted over the past few years at the University of Texas Southwestern Medical Center in Dallas suggest that estrogen acts on the nerves and synapses in that part of the brain that controls memory; thus, when estrogen levels decline, the neurological mechanisms that help you store and retrieve information in your brain may be weakened.

Other research suggests another implied link between estrogen levels and memory. For example, a Canadian study, published in 1992 in a journal called *Psychoneuroendocrinology*, looked at the memory function of women who had become surgically menopausal. Researchers found that before surgery, when estrogen levels were normal, patients' memories were much better than after surgery, when estrogen levels had fallen dramatically. Further, a paper published in a recent issue of the *Journal of the American Medical Association* suggests that while menopausal women undergoing estrogen therapy showed no improvement in cognitive function, of which memory is a key part, that same result did *not* hold true for premenopausal women, leading us to believe that estrogen could improve memory in transitional women. While such memory lapses are not a major problem—and certainly not as uncomfortable as headaches—they can be annoying and, if they occur frequently enough, pretty upsetting.

HEIGHTENED OR DULLED SENSES. Lowered estrogen levels may also affect the way your senses respond to stimuli, and thus lead to another of the NAS: a change in your sensory abilities. Some women report that their senses of smell and taste have gotten either sharper or more dull after thirty-five. For instance, you may discover that while the slightest whiff of something burning used to send you flying into the kitchen, now you barely smell that roast scorching in the oven. Or, maybe you used to love peppery foods but now you find them too hot to tolerate comfortably. If any of these problems strike a familiar chord, you may be suffering from one of the NAS.

As far as I know, no studies have been done to examine whether or not a connection exists between estrogen and the senses in transitional women. However, anecdotal evidence suggests that the senses of taste and smell in menopausal women undergoing estrogen therapy do return to their premenopausal states. This leads me to believe that there may indeed be some sort of association between transitional women's changed senses and their declining estrogen levels.

LOWERED STAMINA. Having less energy and stamina ranks among the most common of the NAS and is often a complaint of transitional women. You just don't seem to have your old get-up-and-go, although blood tests and doctors' examinations reveal nothing wrong.

Frequently, a drop in your energy level can be traced to factors that have nothing to do with declining estrogen or problems with your nervous system. For example, too much stress or a diet rich in fat and protein and deficient in complex carbohydrates (grains, fruits, and vegetables) can reduce your stamina. Many times, however, estrogen, a change in the action of your nerves, and age have an important impact.

Stamina, which is your ability to endure physical stress over long periods of time, centers on two main factors: bone density and muscle strength. We've already discussed estrogen's role in keeping bones strong. But here's how the hormone influences muscle strength.

When you exercise your muscles—not just during a workout, but through everyday activities—you accumulate lactic acid in your blood vessels. A certain amount of this is perfectly normal. But when there is inadequate oxygen being carried to the muscles and surrounding tissue, lactic acid accumulates at a much faster rate, which causes muscle pain and fatigue and prevents you from going on. Estrogen helps keep those blood vessels carrying oxygen to your muscles clear, thereby preventing, or at least dramatically slowing, this buildup of lactic acid. A decrease in estrogen during the transitional years, therefore, can hamper this oxygenation and thus reduce your stamina.

Additionally, estrogen stimulation at the synapse of the nerves is reduced as the hormone levels decline, which can cause your muscles to begin to lose some strength as you exercise them over a period of time. Aging, too, can weaken the action of nerves on muscles and contribute to the loss of muscle strength and endurance. When you compound these physiological changes with the fairly frenetic life-style that often marks the transitional years, you can understand why total physical stamina declines. Thus, you tire a bit more easily and need a little more rest than you used to, particularly as you reach your late thirties and early forties.

How to remedy NAS.

NAS doesn't necessarily *require* treatment. The symptoms are not life-threatening or dangerous in any way. If they are infrequent, mild, and not particularly bothersome, there's nothing you need to do. In fact, there's really nothing you *can* do to improve one of the NAS—that is, a change in your sense of taste or smell. True, estrogen might help, but if a sensory change is your only symptom, I believe the risk of estrogen therapy far outweighs any benefit. And I am not aware of any other tactics that can help you regain total sensory function. However, if any of the other NAS I've discussed make you uncomfortable or disrupt your life in any way, try these strategies.

To relieve headaches.

- *Over-the-counter medications.* Nonsteroidal drugs such as aspirin, Motrin, Advil, Midol, and Nuprin can help reduce inflammation in and around the brain and help soothe headache pain. Avoid preparations that contain caffeine, such as Excedrin Extra Strength or Anacin Maximum Strength.
- *Antihistamines.* An allergic response that releases histamines in the brain can lead to headaches. If allergies are

your problem, antihistamines may help your headaches disappear. They often cause drowsiness and lethargy, so don't take them when you need your wits about you. Of course, if you're getting persistent allergy headaches, consulting a professional allergist is a wise idea.

• *Estrogen Supplemental Therapy (EST)*. If none of the above remedies help, talk with your doctor about EST. Small amounts of estrogen taken the first ten days of your cycle should bring relief.

To enhance your memory.

As I mentioned earlier, estrogen therapy may help to improve your memory. If, however, occasional memory lapses are your only complaint, *I would not prescribe estrogen as a remedy* for the same reason I would not recommend it to restore your sense of smell or taste—the risks clearly outweigh the benefits. Instead, if memory problems are bothersome, try the following tactics.

• *Memory-enhancing games.* Scientists hypothesize that whenever you learn anything, you store it in a cubbyhole in your brain. To recall the information, a signal is sent along your brain pathways to that cubbyhole and the datum is retrieved—you "remember" your first grade teacher's name, the sum of 2 + 2, the farthest planet from the earth. But as you get older, those brain pathways weaken, and unless you use them persistently they don't function as well, a situation that can result in short-term memory lapses.

Memory-enhancing games, particularly card games such as bridge, pinochle, or poker, force you to exercise your brain and thus keep your memory in better shape. Adopting techniques that help compensate for short-term lapses is also helpful. Simply posting a reminder in a conspicuous place, for instance, or writing a list of the things you need to remember can help. So can associations. If you can't remember people's names, for example, next time you meet someone new try linking his or her name with an idea that will trigger your memory. For instance, you might remember "Skip" because he is a marathon runner.

- *Stress-reducing mechanisms.* When your pace is too frantic and there's just too much on your mind, your memory can slip. In that case, such holistic techniques as yoga, massage, guided imagery, and meditation can soothe your mind, body, and spirit—and let you relax.
- *Mild stimulants.* Certain mild stimulants such as coffee, tea, and cola can sharpen short-term memory, although the caffeine can cause problems in other ways, as we've discussed in earlier chapters.
- *Antidepressants.* Although I would not prescribe or recommend antidepressants as a remedy for memory complaints, if you're already taking such new antidepressants as Paxil and Zoloft for an emotional problem, you may find your short-term memory improving.

To increase your stamina.

To cure a temporary downturn in your energy level, try mild stimulants such as tea. Coffee's okay, too—*if* you keep it down to fewer than two cups a day. But in the long run, the best way to keep up your energy level is to follow my ten-point plan on page 30.

A Recommendation to Take Action

If the problems associated with NAS are getting you down, take action. That's what forty-four-year-old Betty Ann did. Betty Ann holds a very responsible but stressful position working as a magazine editor. When she came to see me for her regular checkup last year, she complained that she didn't have the stamina she needed to get through her very busy schedule and that she had started getting frequent headaches.

I ran a routine blood test to rule out any chemical imbalances, but the results were perfectly normal. Since she'd mentioned that the headaches were particularly severe on the right side of her head, I was worried that her complaint might be a more involved neurological problem, so I referred her to a neurologist. Once again, though, test results revealed no difficulties.

Then I noticed something else: Betty Ann seemed to be having some difficulty remembering simple things, such as the name of the neurologist I'd sent her to and where his office was located. When I asked Betty Ann if she'd noticed any problems with her memory, she said that she had been having some trouble with little things recently, such as misplacing files at the office or forgetting where she'd left the coffee cup she'd set down minutes before. Since we had already ruled out any serious problems with her brain and blood chemistry, I began to suspect that her reduced energy, headaches, and memory slips were NAS.

After explaining my ideas about NAS to Betty Ann, I made a few recommendations: first, I suggested she take a vacation from work—something she hadn't done for two years! Additionally, I encouraged her to attend relaxation seminars and stress management sessions. I also urged her to revise her eating habits—which had included lots of sugary snacks—and follow my guidelines for a balanced diet. Finally, I asked her to make another appointment to see me in two months.

When Betty Ann returned, she was much happier. She said her stamina had improved and her memory seemed much better. She was still getting headaches, although they'd gone from three or four severe ones each week to one or two mild headaches a month. Since she was so pleased with her progress, we agreed that taking more aggressive measures was not necessary.

If you believe you are suffering from one or more of the NAS, try some of the simpler remedies I've offered first; if they don't help, ask your doctor for more aggressive tactics, such as medication. But here's what's most important: don't assume you have to live with the discomfort, embarrassment, or pain that NAS can cause. The transitional years can—and should—be a time to enjoy your best and healthiest self.

9

The Thyroid: Outsmarting a Midlife Imposter

- Signs and Symptoms of Thyroid Disorders
- How the Thyroid Works
- Diagnosing Thyroid Disorders
- Treating Your Underactive Thyroid
- Treating Your Overactive Thyroid
- Are You at Risk for Future Thyroid Problems?

Suddenly one day, a familiar but alarmingly middle-aged-looking woman stares back at you from your mirror. All the signs are there: the puffy eyes, the dry skin, the brittle hair. Just as bad, you feel sluggish and run-down even though you seem to sleep more than usual. You've been having trouble concentrating and remembering things lately. You've been constipated, feel cold all the time, and have put on a few pounds even though you haven't been eating more than usual. "Well," you say to yourself, "I guess it's all part of middle age. Better get used to it." Right?

Wrong.

While some of these problems do tend to surface as you begin to approach menopause, they're not inevitable. If you take good care of yourself, it could be years before any of these changes appear.

You need to know, however, that if your thyroid malfunctions, it can trigger many problems associated with midlife. In fact, thyroid symptoms are such savvy masqueraders of common age-related woes—skillfully mimicking a number of illnesses, including clinical depression, heart disease, arthritis, even cancer—that they frequently fool even doctors.

What's even more disturbing is that thyroid disorders occur with alarming frequency among transitional women. Millions of women between the ages of thirty-six and fifty show signs of a failing thyroid, according to the Thyroid Foundation of America, a patient information organization based in Boston. By age fifty, fully one in ten women suffers from hypothyroidism, an underactive thyroid—and half of them don't even know it! (Yes, there *is* a link between declining estrogen and thyroid function, as I'll discuss shortly.)

Although no definitive statistics on hyperthyroidism (overactive thyroid) exist, a spokesperson for the National Thyroid Foundation says that it is a far less common problem than hypothyroidism. However, the foundation does report that hyperthyroidism strikes women three to eight times more often than men.

SIGNS AND SYMPTOMS OF THYROID DISORDERS

While a blood test is the only accurate way to tell for sure whether or not your thyroid is working correctly, certain symptoms can tip you off to a problem. Read through the two checklists that follow and put an X next to any statement that applies to you. If you mark four or more, it's probably time to get your thyroid checked.

SYMPTOM CHECKLIST FOR HYPOTHYROIDISM

___ I feel sluggish and tired a great deal of the time.
___ I'm feeling down and depressed.
___ I'm gaining weight, even though I'm eating less.
___ I'm sleeping more than usual.
___ I'm often constipated.
___ I have some difficulty with concentration and memory.
___ I'm less interested in sex than usual.
___ My hair feels dry and brittle.
___ I haven't had a period for several months.
___ My periods have been irregular, with heavy bleeding.
___ My voice sounds deeper and huskier than normal.
___ I feel stiff when I get out of bed in the morning.
___ My skin is dry and scaly.
___ I feel cold even when others around me are comfortable.
___ The collars on my blouses feel tighter than usual.
___ I can't seem to get pregnant.
___ My nails are brittle and growing more slowly than usual.
___ I'm getting puffy around my eyes.

— My cholesterol level has gone up, even though my diet is unchanged.
— I seem to have become slightly hard of hearing lately.

SYMPTOM CHECKLIST FOR HYPERTHYROIDISM

— I have a lot of nervous energy; I can't seem to sit still.
— Every so often, my heart starts pounding for no apparent reason.
— My pulse seems more rapid than usual.
— My favorite blouse seems tighter around the neck.
— I have trouble sleeping at night.
— I sweat more than usual.
— My eyes seem to be bulging slightly.
— I've been losing weight and I don't understand why.
— I've had diarrhea a lot lately.
— The heat bothers me much more than it used to.
— I'm hungrier than normal.
— I get irritable or moody more often than usual.
— My menstrual periods are scanty.
— I've had several bouts of indigestion lately.
— My ankles are swollen.

If you think you may have a thyroid problem, here's what you should *not* do: worry. We have very effective treatments for thyroid disorders. Here's what you *should* do: talk with your doctor. He or she can perform a few simple tests (I'll describe them shortly) that can confirm your suspicion or set your mind at ease. To understand the importance of correcting a thyroid disorder, you need to understand why the thyroid has such far-reaching impact on your overall health and well-being.

How the Thyroid Works

Located at the base of your neck, and shaped like a butterfly with its wings extended around your windpipe, the thyroid gland weighs barely an ounce, but it's a giant when it comes to biological activity. This gland is the chief regulator of your body's metabolism, the CEO of all physical and chemical changes that take place in your body.

The thyroid regulates nearly every tissue and organ by releasing certain hormones into your blood. The thyroid makes two hormones: *triiodothyronine* (T_3), the active hormone; and *thyroxine* (T_4), which is converted into T_3 after it's released from the gland. The thyroid also serves as a warehouse for the hormones it makes, which is why even if your thyroid were suddenly to stop producing hormones, your body wouldn't notice the difference for a week or longer, until the gland had depleted its reserves.

Normally, the thyroid makes, stores, and releases just enough hormones to keep your body running smoothly. It does so with help from the pituitary gland, located at the base of your brain; this gland sends a modest amount of another hormone, called thyroid stimulating hormone (TSH), to the thyroid gland to help keep it functioning properly.

The pituitary continuously checks your blood to see how much T_3 is present. If there's a dip in your T_3 level, it sends more TSH to the thyroid to stimulate the release of additional hormone. If there's a high level of T_3 in your blood, the pituitary holds back on its release of some TSH. Usually this system of checks and balances works beautifully, but when the thyroid is malfunctioning, there is nothing the pituitary can do to remedy the situation. This is why individuals with hypothyroidism have high TSH but low thyroid hormone levels; the pituitary is sending out lots of TSH to try to get the underactive thyroid to work harder and put out more thyroid hormone. This also explains why the opposite holds true for people with hyperthyroidism; they have excessive T_3 levels and low TSH.

Sex hormones and your thyroid.

The pituitary isn't the only gland that works together with the thyroid. Years ago, when I was a resident at the Woman's Medical College of Pennsylvania, now the Medical College of Pennsylvania, I published, with Dr. Mary Dratman, what has become a landmark paper showing a close relationship between the ovaries and the thyroid. These glands support and sustain each other through the hormones they release. Most important for transitional women is the fact that when estrogen levels decline, the thyroid gland may falter. As estrogen levels begin to decline after age thirty-five, your chances for thyroid troubles increase. Similarly, when the thyroid stops working properly, the ovaries may malfunction.

Our research also shed some light on the idea that a number of significant women's health troubles are really thyroid disorders in disguise. In fact, any of the following are reason enough to get your thyroid checked.

- *You can't seem to get pregnant.* Thyroid disorders, particularly hypothyroidism, are a major but very treatable cause of infertility. The reason is that an underactive thyroid upsets the delicate mechanism that controls ovulation, preventing an egg from being released at the proper time.
- *You're suffering from postpartum blues.* You've undoubtedly read or heard a good deal about postpartum depression, a problem that affects up to one quarter of all

The Thyroid: Outsmarting a Midlife Imposter

new mothers. What you may not know, however, is that a thyroid problem is often the real culprit.

Researchers estimate that about 10 percent of women suffering from postpartum depression actually have "postpartum thyroiditis," an inflammation of the thyroid gland that can occur within six weeks to three months after delivery, completely unbeknownst to the new mother.

We're not exactly sure why this inflammation occurs in some women but not in others. One popular hypothesis involves the immune system. After delivery, some women begin to produce harmful autoimmune antibodies that seem to be stirred up by a previous viral infection within the thyroid. They attack the gland, causing it to become swollen and inflamed.

In its early stage, postpartum thyroiditis may cause temporary hyperthyroidism, as thyroid hormone leaks out of the swollen gland. But this overactivity is brief, often causes no symptoms, and thus goes unnoticed. A few weeks later, however, as the damage silently continues, the new mother can develop hypothyroidism; then she begins to suffer from such symptoms as fatigue, depression, and poor concentration. Happily, though, a short course of treatment usually clears the problem. Only when damage is moderate to severe might you need to consider long-term thyroid hormone replacement therapy.

- *Your sex drive stalls out.* In my years of practice, I've treated so many women with thyroid disorders who also complained of losing their interest in sex that I decided to conduct a formal research study. The findings, published in the *Journal of Clinical Practice in Sexuality* in 1992, show that nearly 90 percent of women with hypothyroidism, and roughly half of those with hyperthyroidism, experience a loss of sexual enjoyment. Their problems run the gamut, from feeling too tired to make love to experiencing painful intercourse because of a decrease in vaginal secretions. On a brighter note, I also found that these sexual troubles usually vanish after we identify and treat the underlying thyroid disorder.

- *You're having annoying menstrual problems.* If you have hypothyroidism, your menstrual flow may become much lighter and the intervals between your periods may lengthen. With hyperthyroidism, you may have much longer, heavier, and more frequent periods. Because transitional women tend to develop menstrual irregularities anyway as they approach menopause, many doctors blame menstrual changes on aging rather than what could be the real culprit: a malfunctioning thyroid. Make sure you get your thyroid tested before consenting to a D&C or a hysterectomy to diagnose or correct menstrual troubles. In fact, it's best to get your thyroid checked if you have *any* menstrual problems, particularly if they occur along with any of the other symptoms of thyroid trouble.

- *You're suffering early menopausal symptoms.* Hypothyroidism can sometimes mimic the symptoms of menopause, as forty-year-old Marcella discovered. She came in for her annual checkup convinced that she was entering menopause. Marcella had gone four months without a period and suffered from vaginal dryness, which she knew were both common symptoms of estrogen deficiency. She was understandably upset about her symptoms, not only because she felt she was growing old before her time, but also because she and her husband wanted to have a second child and she feared she was infertile.

I did a routine blood study to measure the levels of Marcella's reproductive and thyroid hormones. The lab results revealed that she wasn't going through early menopause be-

The Thyroid: Outsmarting a Midlife Imposter

cause her FSH level, which rises sharply after menopause, was perfectly normal. Instead, we found that Marcella's TSH level was very high, indicating that her thyroid was underactive. In her case, severe hypothyroidism had caused her pituitary gland to pump out not only huge amounts of TSH but also another hormone called prolactin. The excess prolactin, in turn, had shut down her ovaries and turned off her menstrual cycles, understandably fooling her into thinking that she was menopausal.

Within two months of treatment with thyroid hormone, Marcella's periods resumed. And one year later, when I saw Marcella again, she was pregnant! She and her husband are now the parents of two healthy, happy kids.

(FYI: Because Marcella was hypothyroid she needed special attention throughout her pregnancy. Even in a healthy woman, pregnancy puts extra demands on the thyroid. Women with hypothyroidism need bimonthly thyroid checkups to ensure that their thyroid hormone levels remain in sync with the changing needs of pregnancy. Left untreated, hypothyroidism can harm a developing fetus; the baby's thyroid may become enlarged and make too much thyroid hormone as if it were trying to help its mother out. Additionally, maternal hypothyroidism heightens the risk of miscarriage.)

Hyperthyroidism can also trick you into thinking you're menopausal. Forty-seven-year-old Patricia is a typical example. She was constantly asking her office mates to turn up the air-conditioning because she always felt so hot and flushed. During those days when her job became particularly stressful, she'd begin to perspire profusely, which made her feel disheveled and self-conscious. When some of her male co-workers began teasing her about having hot flashes, Patricia found her way to my office.

"It's not just that I'm sweating, Bernie," she told me.

"My periods have become very light and I've been very irritable at the office, snapping at colleagues over minor annoyances, which is something I never used to do." Patricia also reported that she'd had frequent bouts of diarrhea and that she'd lost five pounds lately, even though she'd been eating more than normal. She felt her heart racing erratically on occasion, which made her worry that she'd developed a heart problem.

To get at the root of her problems, I did a complete blood workup that included a TSH test. The results revealed good and bad news: her estrogen and FSH levels were normal, so she was not in menopause, but her TSH level was extremely low, a sign that she was hyperthyroid. Further tests showed that Patricia had a form of hyperthyroidism called Graves' disease—the same condition that afflicts former first lady Barbara Bush. As occurs in postpartum thyroiditis, in Graves' disease misguided antibodies attack and damage the thyroid, stimulating it to release too much hormone. I treated Patricia with antithyroid medication and when I next saw her, her symptoms had disappeared and the problem was under control.

Diagnosing Thyroid Disorders

Thyroid disorders can be subtle, so it's a good idea for transitional women to pay close attention to their bodies. If you notice any symptoms that could be thyroid-related, tell your doctor. He or she will probably not be able to diagnose a thyroid disorder based only on your symptoms, but blood work usually pinpoints the problem.

Your doctor will begin your thyroid evaluation by taking your medical history and noting your complaints. He'll check your blood pressure (hyperthyroidism raises blood pressure, hypothyroidism lowers it), and your pulse (hyperthyroidism speeds up your pulse, hypothyroidism slows it). Your doctor will look at your eyes for such signs as bulging, which could indicate hyperthyroidism, or slower lid movements, which could signal hypothyroidism. Then, the doctor will check your reflexes; the knee-jerk response is faster and more intense than normal with hyperthyroidism, and slower and more sluggish than normal with hypothyroidism.

Next, your physician will check the gland itself by palpating, or feeling, it for any enlargement or abnormality. A healthy thyroid feels relatively smooth and soft, not hard or lumpy. An enlarged thyroid, called a goiter, can occur in either hyperthyroidism or hypothyroidism and is often the first sign of a problem.

If your doctor suspects a problem, he or she will take a blood sample to measure your thyroid function. The thyroid hormones T_3 and T_4 can be measured with a variety of tests. Because hormone levels vary considerably from individual to individual, however, measurement alone may not offer a clear diagnosis. To confirm the existence of a problem, you should have a test called a "sensitive TSH assay." Since TSH level is an effective indicator of thyroid function, the test offers great accuracy.

As I've already noted, if your TSH is high and your thyroid hormones are low, you probably have hypothyroidism. If TSH is low or absent and the thyroid hormones are high, it's a good bet you have hyperthyroidism. If both TSH and thyroid hormones are normal, your thyroid is probably functioning just fine. Occasionally, however, the lab findings are not very clear-cut. Sometimes I see women who have definite symptoms of hypothyroidism but whose TSH levels are in the gray zone between normal and high. In these cases, I treat them to relieve the symptoms, then recommend close follow-up care to see if any more problems arise. If they improve with thyroid medication and show no further symptoms, the diagnosis is confirmed.

Further diagnostic tests.

Both hypothyroidism and hyperthyroidism have many causes, so if your checkup suggests a thyroid problem your doctor will ask you to take a few additional tests to pinpoint the trouble as specifically as possible. For instance, your thyroid may have lumps or nodules. While these are usually harmless, they must always be looked at more closely to rule out the possibility of cancer. Additional thyroid tests include:

- *Thyroid ultrasound.* This painless, fifteen-minute test uses sound waves to take a picture of your thyroid. To perform the test, a technician will move a small instrument called a transducer over your neck. The transducer beams sound waves at your thyroid, then picks up the reflected waves as they bounce off the gland. The information is fed into a computer, which analyzes it and displays a picture of your thyroid on a television screen. Ultrasound can reveal an enlarged thyroid, pinpoint the size and location of fluid-filled cysts, and reveal solid benign or malignant tumors.
- *Radioactive iodine uptake test.* Because the thyroid uses iodine to produce its hormones, the rate at which your thyroid absorbs iodine is a sound indicator of how active your thyroid is. You'll be asked to drink a tasteless solution containing a miniscule amount of radioactive iodine. At six and at twenty-four hours later, the amount of radioactive iodine in your thyroid is scanned with a radiation detector. If you have hyperthyroidism, nearly all of the radioactive iodine is absorbed, or taken up, by the overactive gland. If you have

hypothyroidism or postpartum thyroiditis, little or none is absorbed.

- *Thyroid scan.* Particularly helpful for screening tumors, the thyroid scan is usually done at the time of the uptake test. This procedure involves connecting the radiation detector to a scanner, which creates a picture of the distribution of radioactive iodine within the thyroid. If the iodine is widely diffused throughout the gland, the entire thyroid is probably overactive. If the iodine is concentrated in a few nodules, your hyperthyroidism may be confined to these "hot spots," which may, in fact, be tumors.

Treating Your Underactive Thyroid

Happily, the best treatment for hypothyroidism is a simple one: taking a pill made of synthetic thyroxine (T_4) once a day to replace the natural hormone you require but that your thyroid can no longer produce sufficiently. Your doctor will work carefully with you to adjust the dose up or down until you find the amount that works best for you. (NOTE: If you're taking estrogen, make sure you let your doctor know; thyroid medication interacts with estrogen supplements.) Thyroxine replacement therapy is safe, inexpensive, and fast-acting—within a few weeks, you'll be back to normal. Your energy will be replenished, your fertility will be restored, even your puffy eyes will smooth out.

What you need to know about taking thyroxine.

Millions of women take thyroxine every day; it ranks among the top ten prescription drugs in America. Although thyroxine is a safe form of therapy, supplying what your body would ordinarily make on its own, it's still medicine and must be taken with care. To take thyroxine safely, follow these simple tips:

- *Take your medication at the same time every day.* The whole idea of thyroxine replacement therapy is to maintain a constant, steady level of thyroid hormone in your blood, just as a normal thyroid gland would do. If you forget and skip a dose, which you're more likely to do if you don't take the pill at the same time each day, you defeat the purpose of the medication because the level of hormone will vary.
- *Take your medication in the morning.* Like a cup of strong coffee, thyroid medication can give your system a bit of a jolt and prevent you from falling asleep if you take it too late in the day. That's why I recommend taking your pill in the morning. If you have to take it twice a day, take a greater dosage in the morning and just enough to maintain yourself later in the day.
- *Take only the amount prescribed.* An overzealous patient of mine once decided that if a little thyroxine could make her feel more energetic, more would give her extraordinary get-up-and-go. So she took an extra half tablet every day. Her plan backfired. A month or so later, she burst into my office complaining that she couldn't sleep at night and that she had persistent diarrhea and heart palpitations. Apparently, she'd taken so much added thyroxine that she made herself hyperthyroid! Luckily, she'd done no permanent damage. When she went back to the dosage I'd prescribed, she felt fine again.
- *Get your thyroid checked every six months.* Even if your treatment has you feeling terrific, make sure you have a thyroid evaluation twice a year. At your age, your thyroid can change and your doctor may need to compensate for these changes by readjusting your dosage. You should

also alert your doctor to any new symptoms or problems that appear. For instance, if you start feeling jittery or overheated, you may be taking more thyroxine than you need.

- *Take thyroxine for a thyroid problem only.* In some cases, women with perfectly normal thyroids are being given thyroid medication to control their weight (since it revs up your metabolism), to relieve swelling and bloat, or to treat lethargy. I disagree with these uses of thyroid medication and would caution you against all of them. Taking thyroid hormone when your gland's working fine can cause what is essentially drug-induced hyperthyroidism and trigger all the problems we've just discussed.

Treating Your Overactive Thyroid

Today, several treatment options are available for people with hyperthyroidism. Which one is right for you depends largely on your age, the type of hyperthyroidism you suffer from, and whether or not you're troubled by other medical conditions. Here are the best and most widely-used remedies:

Drug therapy.

Medications that prevent the thyroid from making too much thyroid hormone do wonders for people with hyperthyroidism. Most likely, your doctor will prescribe either methimazole (Tapazole) or propylthiouracil (PTU) pills taken daily for a period of six to twelve months. These drugs can cause some drowsiness and minor lethargy; rarely, they can cause agranulocytosis, a blood disease. Most of the time, however, this form of therapy is safe and restores normal hormone balance within a couple of months.

Radioactive iodine therapy.

If drug treatment fails, I sometimes recommend radioactive iodine therapy. Although it sounds kind of scary and dangerous, it's usually quite safe. You're given a capsule or a drink of water containing radioactive iodine. After being swallowed, the "radioiodine" is rapidly absorbed by the overactive thyroid cells, which are destroyed by the radiation, so less thyroid hormone is produced. The radioactivity disappears from your body within days.

You should *not* undergo radioactive iodine therapy while you are pregnant. The radiation can adversely affect a developing fetus. Transitional women planning to have a baby within the next few years should also beware. I've conducted some studies that show that iodine can be absorbed by the ovaries as well as the thyroid. This means developing ova could be affected. For this reason—and I know I'm more conservative than many other doctors on this issue—I do *not* recommend this therapy to women over thirty-five who plan to become pregnant within the next few years.

Surgery.

Occasionally, removing all or part of the thyroid is the best solution for hyperthyroidism. If only a single lump or nodule within the thyroid is producing too much hormone, your surgeon can take out just that small part of the gland. If the entire gland is overactive, which is more often the case, you'll need a total thyroidectomy, removal of the whole gland. Sometimes, however, your surgeon can leave a small portion of the thyroid intact—just enough to produce adequate amounts of thyroid hormone. Depending on how much of the gland is left after surgery, you may need subsequent thyroid replacement therapy.

A final cautionary note: treatment for hyperthyroidism sometimes can lead to hypothyroidism, so if you're under treatment for an overactive thyroid, it's important that you get annual thyroid checkups for the rest of your life.

ARE YOU AT RISK FOR FUTURE THYROID PROBLEMS?

Because thyroid problems are relatively common in transitional women, it's important that you get your thyroid tested periodically. For most women, I recommend getting a thyroid evaluation every two years, starting at age thirty-six, even if you have no troublesome symptoms. That way, you can detect a problem at an early stage when it's easier to treat. Finding a problem early on also lessens the chances that you'll be duped into thinking your symptoms indicate early menopause, heart trouble, depression, or other conditions with symptoms similar to those of a malfunctioning thyroid. Your primary care doctor or gynecologist can do the checkup, which consists of two steps: first, feeling the thyroid manually to make sure that it is not enlarged; and second, taking blood and sending it to the lab for thyroid function analysis.

I recommend annual thyroid checkups to transitional women whose family histories or past experiences put them at higher risk of thyroid problems. If any of the following pertain to you, you are at higher risk:

- *Radiation treatment during childhood.* During the heyday of the atomic age in the forties and fifties, healthy kids were often treated with head or neck irradiation for anything from enlarged tonsils to teenage acne. Some babies were given neck irradiation to shrink an enlarged thymus gland, a part of the immune system.

We now know that these treatments were unnecessary, but unfortunately, today we're still experiencing the fallout. When the head or neck of these children was irradiated, in many cases so, too, was the nearby thyroid gland. Doctors now know that exposing the thyroid to external radiation during childhood can lead to such thyroid problems as hypothyroidism or tumors in adulthood. In fact, childhood radiation treatment is a leading cause of adult thyroid cancer. (TAKE NOTE: Only external radiation *treatments* increase your risk of cancer, not diagnostic X-rays or radioactive iodine therapy.)

If you think or know you had head or neck radiation therapy as a child, be sure to have annual thyroid checkups regardless of whether you notice any of the typical symptoms of a thyroid disorder. It's the only way to catch silent abnormalities before they cause any permanent harm. Don't worry, though. As we've already discussed, thyroid problems are treatable. Even if your doctor finds a malignancy, you should know that most thyroid cancers can be completely cured with early detection and treatment. Because thyroid cancers usually grow slowly, early detection gives you time to consider your treatment options carefully.

- *A family history of thyroid problems.* Several thyroid conditions, including Graves' disease, are inherited. So a family history could heighten your risk for a problem. On the other hand, just because a family member has thyroid trouble doesn't mean you'll have the same fate. You just need to be a bit more vigilant about regular thyroid checkups.

- *Premature hair and skin changes.* Premature gray, patchy hair loss on your scalp, and painless white spots on your hands, arms, or neck have been linked to a genetic predisposition to hypothyroidism. If you have any of these conditions, you should get your thyroid checked at least once a year—more, if your doctor recommends it.
- *You live in a "goiter belt."* If you live in an area where there's not much iodine in the water or ground, you're at risk for thyroid problems. You'll need to use iodized salt in your diet and to see your doctor regularly to make sure your thyroid is healthy. Sections of the country where people may be at risk include the Great Lakes region, the western plains, and such mountainous areas as the Appalachians, Adirondacks, and Rockies. (Not sure if the town you live in is affected? Although people who live in goiter belts usually know it—it's widely publicized—you can call your local health department to double-check.)
- *You're taking lithium.* Lithium, often prescribed to control severe mood swings, can cause the thyroid to become underactive or overactive. That doesn't mean you shouldn't take this drug. On the contrary, lithium is quite safe, as long as you get regular thyroid checkups to spot early signs of trouble.

Because a malfunctioning thyroid is not the first thought in the minds of health care providers faced with any number of symptoms in patients in their transitional years, you need to become more attuned to the possibility yourself. If you suspect a problem, insist that your thyroid be checked. When thyroid disorders are left undiagnosed and are therefore untreated, the symptoms can become unpleasant—and could well prevent you from enjoying the best quality of life available.

10

Beating Serious Illness

- Heart Disease
- Problems with Arteries and Veins
- Pulmonary Problems
- Gynecological Cancers
- Cancer Treatment After Thirty-Five

Most women go through their transitional years without ever having to face a serious illness, but not everyone is that lucky. As unpleasant as it may be to consider, the risk for certain medical problems begins to increase once you pass your mid-thirties. Specifically, problems with the heart, veins and arteries, breathing apparatus, even cancer, are more likely to occur in women over thirty-five than they are in younger women.

But there's good news, too: we know so much more about these ailments today than we used to that doctors like myself can not only help you cut your risk of developing a serious illness, but also can detect, effectively treat, and in some cases cure an illness before it ever has a chance to harm the quality of your life. But the first move is yours. Familiarizing yourself with these illnesses will help you work knowledgeably and proactively with your doctor to stay in the best possible health.

Heart Disease

Recent studies have put us all on the alert: they've suggested that women may not be receiving the same attention—or treatment—for heart disease as men. For instance, most of the studies on cardiac disease have excluded women. When researchers at Brigham and Women's Hospital in Massachusetts reviewed more than two hundred studies on heart disease published between 1990 and 1991, for example, they found that women were highly underrepresented; in fact, fewer than 20 percent of the study subjects were women.

Another fact, noted at the January 1992 conference of the National Heart, Lung and Blood Institute on "Cardiovascular Health and Disease in Women": doctors have tended not to take women's complaints of chest pain as seriously as men's. This is due to a misperception that heart disease is not as dangerous a problem for women as it is for men.

I find this gender bias extremely distressing because heart disease is the number one killer of American women. Although women tend to fear breast cancer the most, heart attacks kill about six times as many women, according to the American Heart Association.

True, young women aren't at high risk for heart trouble. Between the ages of twenty-five and thirty-five, women develop heart disease at one third the rate men of the same age do. After age thirty-six, however, that difference starts to dwindle. In the latter part of their transitional years women are still at lower risk than men, but the gap has begun to narrow. By age seventy-five, both sexes are equally likely to have heart trouble. (It may well be that women have been underrepresented in research on heart disease because most studies and clinical trials exclude the elderly, the age group in which women's risk reaches its highest level.)

Here's what's most important for transitional women to understand: although you're not as likely to develop cardiac disease as older, menopausal women are, you're not risk-free, either. Most important, certain factors that are within your control can heighten your chance for a heart problem right now and dramatically raise your risk for trouble in the future.

Risk factors associated with cardiac disease.

DECLINING ESTROGEN. We believe that women over age thirty-six have a higher risk for heart disease because of our old friend, estrogen. More specifically, studies have linked this powerful hormone with harmful changes in cholesterol levels.

As you probably know, cholesterol, the fatlike substance found in animal tissue, consists of two types of lipoprotein: high density lipoprotein (HDL) and low density lipoprotein (LDL). HDL is "the good stuff" because it carries cholesterol away from the tissues and to the liver, where it can be excreted from the body. High levels of HDL are linked with low incidence of cardiac disease. LDL, on the other hand, is "the bad stuff" because it's the main carrier of cholesterol in the blood. High levels of LDL seem to promote cholesterol buildup on artery walls, which can lead to atherosclerosis, narrowing of the arteries.

The reason estrogen is so important is that it seems to

raise the level of HDL while lowering LDL, thus protecting women in their peak reproductive years—when estrogen levels are strong—from cardiac disease. But as estrogen begins to decrease in the transitional years, the hormone's protective action diminishes and potentially puts you at greater risk for heart disease. The same phenomenon occurs if for any reason you have your ovaries removed; the sudden elimination of estrogen could make you more vulnerable to cardiac problems.

Recently, I've become involved in more estrogen research with Drs. Jay Roberts and Dave Snyder at the Medical College of Pennsylvania. Our work with aging female rodents and rabbits whose estrogen is decreasing has revealed another possible connection between estrogen and cardiac disease. In our test animals, low estrogen levels appear to affect the nerves of the heart, possibly causing irregularities of the heartbeat. Since these irregularities may be precursors to heart disease, the drop in estrogen *during the transitional years and thereafter* may leave the heart more vulnerable to problems.

IRON.   Still another theory centers on estrogen's indirect effect on iron. A Finnish study, published in the *American Heart Association* journal, shows that men with high levels of iron in their bodies were more likely to have heart attacks than men with normal levels. The reason, these researchers believe, is that iron increases the risk of heart attack by increasing the formation of free radicals. These free radicals in turn interact with LDL cholesterol in a way that promotes the buildup of plaque on arterial walls, leading to atherosclerosis and ultimately heart attack. High levels of stored iron may also weaken the heart muscle and worsen the effects of any heart attack that does occur.

Scientists hypothesize, then, that since estrogen triggers

menstruation, which carries iron away in monthly blood flow, keeping iron levels from getting very high, menstruation (and, indirectly, estrogen) protects women from heart disease. As estrogen decreases and menstruation becomes less regular in the transitional years, iron stores may begin to accumulate and your risk for heart trouble may begin to increase.

One more point: increasing androgen levels in the transitional years may also make cardiac problems more likely. These hormones raise LDL levels and lower HDL levels, which is why scientists believe they may be tied to greater risk for heart disease.

HYPERTENSION (HIGH BLOOD PRESSURE). Blood pressure literally means the force with which blood courses through your arteries. Two types of pressure are measured: systolic, the pressure created by the contraction of the heart muscle; and diastolic, the pressure between beats that indicates the resistance of all the small arteries in the body. The blood pressure of a healthy transitional woman should be somewhere between 110 and 120 (systole) over between 70 and 80 (diastole). Of course, these numbers vary from person to person, but if your pressure reaches 145 or greater systole and 90 or greater diastole, you may suffer from hypertension and should seek medical advice.

A high diastole reading is actually more worrisome than a high systole because it represents the resting level of your heart. If your heart cannot rest enough between pumps, it will be under greater and more constant stress.

Hypertension is often caused by atherosclerosis, a potentially life-threatening condition in which fatty deposits called plaque build up within the arteries, narrowing them and therefore reducing blood flow to the brain and raising your risk for stroke, or cerebral vascular accident (CVA).

When plaque accumulates, it can also throw off a blood clot with potentially dire consequences.

Another, albeit less serious, problem is that hypertension tends to make you tired, which means you'll be less willing to strengthen your heart through exercise. What's more, too little activity could lead to excessive weight gain, another risk factor for cardiac trouble.

OBESITY. If you're 25 percent over your ideal weight, you're at higher risk for heart disease. (If you're not sure what your ideal weight should be, flip back to the weight chart on page 38.) The reason is twofold: first, your heart has to work harder to tote around those excess pounds; second, the extra body fat can lead to higher, and potentially harmful, cholesterol levels.

SMOKING. People who smoke are four times more likely to die from a heart attack than those who don't. If you don't smoke but you live with someone who does, you're three times more likely to have a heart attack than someone who lives with a nonsmoker.

Here's why. Inhaled tobacco smoke constricts your blood vessels, making your heart work harder to move blood throughout your body. Smoking also damages the lungs, decreasing their oxygen capacity, which forces your heart to pump harder to move more blood into your lungs for use by the rest of your body. When your heart is overworked like that, it can begin to pump irregularly, causing breathing difficulties, chest pain, blackouts, and, possibly, a heart attack.

DIABETES. Diabetes is a strong precursor of cardiovascular problems. Diabetic women—even those who have not yet gone through menopause—suffer from atherosclerosis at nearly the same rate as men. The reason is insulin. In healthy individuals, insulin breaks down carbohydrates for the body to use as energy. If there isn't enough insulin in the body, as is true with diabetics, carbohydrates are converted to fat, which can clog up the blood vessels and interfere with blood flow.

Diabetics who are able to get their blood sugar levels completely under control can lower their risk for cardiovascular disease. But even with injected insulin, it's very hard to keep blood sugar levels stable; instead, they tend to go up and down. When sugar levels are on the upswing, the risk for heart problems increases.

Keeping your heart healthy.

There's lots you can start doing right away to cut your chances for heart disease now and in the future. Here are a few simple but significant guidelines.

GET A THOROUGH CHECKUP. Every transitional woman should have a yearly physical exam that includes not only blood pressure and pulse checks but also routine blood studies, which will reveal important information about her heart, liver, and kidneys. If you're forty or over, biannual electrocardiograms (EKGs) are also important. But beware: some doctors tend to ignore slight abnormalities in EKG results because they simply assume women, particularly premenopausal women, aren't at risk. They may also downplay abnormal findings because they know that breasts make it harder to place electrodes properly to get the most reliable reading. If your EKG results turn up abnormal in any way, it's best to see a cardiologist for a further workup. He or she will probably do an echocardiogram (ultrasound of the heart) and, possibly, a positron emission tomography

(PET) test, a scanning procedure that is capable of producing an accurate picture of even slight heart damage in women.

LOWER YOUR CHOLESTEROL. A healthy transitional woman should have a combined cholesterol count of under 200, with LDL under 130 and HDL over 50. If your cholesterol reading is way up, try to get it back into line by eating a low-fat diet that includes forty grams of cholesterol-fighting fiber each day. Also, it's wise to increase your intake of vitamins A (beta carotene) and E, since these vitamins, which are antioxidants, may prevent cholesterol buildup and reduce your risk for atherosclerosis.

If your total cholesterol is over 200 and your LDL is 130 or more, your doctor may prescribe medication in addition to recommending a modified diet and vitamins. One of the most popular drugs is Lopid, which decreases fat (triglycerides) and helps to improve your LDL:HDL ratio by increasing HDL. But Lopid has its drawbacks. It should not be taken by patients with gallbladder disease, gallstones, or kidney problems, and it can cause gastrointestinal upset, anemia, skin rashes, and fatigue.

SLIM DOWN. If you haven't done it yet, take a look at the weight levels chart on page 38 to find the right weight for you. If you're more than 10 percent above your best weight, make a conscious effort to work off those extra pounds through a program that stresses changes in long-term exercise and eating habits, not quick weight loss.

KEEP A LID ON STRESS. None of us leads a stress-free life. And thank goodness for that; otherwise, things would be downright boring! But it's important to learn how to stay calm, slow your breathing, and let your body and mind relax. The stress-reduction techniques I recommend include deep breathing, meditation, muscle relaxation, visualization and guided imagery, massage, and yoga. You also might want to try acupuncture, acupressure, hypnosis, or psychotherapy. Medication is my least favorite, but sometimes an astonishingly effective, alternative. (For a fuller explanation of each of these methods, see Chapter Twelve.)

MOVE IT! To keep your heart in good shape, be sure to maintain a moderate aerobic exercise regimen that exercises your cardiovascular system. As I've already discussed, walking, jogging, swimming, dancing, and tennis are all excellent choices.

STOP SMOKING. If you stop smoking now, your risk for heart problems will eventually approach that of a nonsmoker. Specifically, ten years after quitting, the risk of death through heart disease for people who smoked one pack a day or less is almost the same as for people who never smoked, according to the American Heart Association. To give yourself your best shot at quitting successfully, follow these strategies.

1. Since women tend to smoke under stress, choose a time to stop when you're not under unusual pressure at work or home. But don't let waiting for the perfect time to quit prevent you from ever getting started.
2. If you smoke to control your weight, find a smoking-cessation program that also offers advice on nutrition and weight management right from the start. If you get sugar cravings—a common withdrawal symptom for former smokers—satisfy your yearnings with more healthful sweets such as fruit sorbet, nonfat frozen yogurt, or fresh fruit.
3. Try to quit right after, not before, your next period.

Research suggests withdrawal symptoms are aggravated by premenstrual changes.

4. Get support. Women are usually more successful at quitting when they enlist the moral support of a few close friends who cheer them on.

5. Get regular exercise. Maintaining a moderate, regular exercise program helps you keep stress down to manageable levels, eases withdrawal symptoms, and burns up more calories so you're less likely to gain weight even if you find yourself nibbling a bit more.

6. Consider nicotine replacement therapy. Wearing a nicotine patch (such as Nicoderm or Habitrol) for the initial part of your stop-smoking efforts may help you quit more comfortably. Patches work by releasing gradually decreasing amounts of nicotine into your system until eventually your body needs none at all. Another approach: nicotine gum. Some people find chewing progressively smaller amounts of this gum helps reduce their cigarette cravings by weaning them from their nicotine dependency.

Treating cardiac disease.

Entire books have been written on heart disease, but suffice it to say here that most treatments include changes in diet and exercise habits, as well as medications—for instance, various forms of digitalis are given to regulate your heartbeat—and possibly surgery. It's difficult to repair a damaged heart, however, so the most important thing to keep in mind is to be proactive when it comes to caring for your heart. To protect your good health, don't let anyone relegate you to second-class status.

Problems with Arteries and Veins

The vascular system is your personal roadway of arteries that carry oxygenated blood from your heart to your body's tissues, and veins that carry "used" blood back again. When you're young, these roadways are usually open and clear so that your blood can flow through easily. But as you age, so do your blood vessels—and the chances for various roadblocks and potholes increase. Two circulatory problems common in the transitional years are thrombophlebitis and allergic edema.

Thrombophlebitis.

The word *phlebitis* means the inflammation of a vein. When the inflammation is accompanied by the formation of a clot, called a "thrombus," you have thrombophlebitis. In women, clots usually form in the legs and pelvis. A thrombus can block the flow of blood through the vein, preventing "used" blood from returning to your heart.

The vast majority of the time, the problem, while painful, is not life-threatening. When thrombophlebitis develops in deep, interior blood vessels, however, a portion of the clot could break away and move through the veins to your lungs. A blockage in a blood vessel in your lung is called a pulmonary embolism. If one of the large pulmonary vessels is blocked—and this may happen without your ever having any symptoms at all—you could die.

Who is at risk? Women with diabetes, severe varicose veins, or a family history of thrombophlebitis. If you've had several pelvic infections, you are also at higher risk since PID can cause the walls of the blood vessels in the pelvic area to thicken and become inflamed, and the connective tissue around the vessels to form adhesions, all of which can restrict blood flow.

If you're on your feet a lot and/or are very overweight, you're probably at greater risk also. In that case, it would be smart for you to wear support hose or elasticized stockings.

(FYI: If you're in the hospital and confined to your bed for more than a day or so, you should be given tight elasticized surgical stockings to help keep blood clots from forming in your legs.)

TREATING THROMBOPHLEBITIS. Superficial thrombophlebitis is easily treated with frequent periods of rest with your legs elevated since the condition mostly occurs within the legs. Aspirin and such nonsteroidal antiinflammatory drugs as Advil and Motrin often help to relieve inflammation and reduce pain. If the condition was caused by a bacterial infection or a secondary infection occurred, your doctor will probably prescribe an antibiotic.

If you suffer from deep thrombophlebitis, treatment is a lot more aggressive. You may be given such anticoagulants as Heparin—usually taken by injection in a hospital—and Coumadin, a pill taken in a maintenance dose for several months. These medications work to dissolve existing clots and to reduce the chance that any new clots will form.

One more point: if you're susceptible to clots, you've got another reason not to smoke. Smoking promotes their formation.

Allergic edema.

Women ages thirty-five to forty-five are particularly susceptible to angioneurotic edema, an allergic response characterized by large areas of swelling in the subcutaneous tissues (the tissues under the skin), mucous membranes, and, occasionally, certain internal organs, such as the abdominal organs. Often, angioneurotic edema causes uncomfortable swelling of the hands, arms, feet, and legs.

I believe that this allergic condition may also be associated with low levels of estrogen. Here's why. A 1986 study done in Britain and a 1991 study at Michigan State University looked at the relationship between estrogen and the immune system. Both found that high levels of estrogen were associated with a strong, healthy immune response. Conversely, low levels of estrogen would weaken the immune response.

For example, an individual with a normal, healthy immune response can experience a certain amount of swelling in the area where an antigen, or foreign body, is introduced. This swelling is caused by the blood's exuding fluids containing antibodies and other substances to fend off the antigen. But when your immune system is weakened, it does not have the usual antibodies to defend itself. So a compensatory mechanism kicks in; that is, the blood keeps exuding more and more fluid in the hope that eventually enough antibodies will collect in the affected area to resist the antigen. The result is a larger amount of swelling than would appear when the immune system is strong. It is this kind of severe swelling that characterizes angioneurotic edema.

I found more evidence of the link between estrogen and the immune system in research several of my colleagues and I conducted in 1993. When we studied the medical histories of a random sample of women who went through the emergency room, we noticed that those who either had their period or were just about to menstruate—that is, women whose estrogen levels had plunged acutely—tended to have more of this kind of swelling of their extremities, and to have more asthma, another allergic reaction, because their bodies were unable to resist whatever antigen had affected them.

Of course, how an individual's immune system responds to an allergen is complicated by the fact that people vary in their sensitivities and that what may trigger an allergic response in one person may not in another. Simply put, I may eat tuna fish and blow up like a balloon whereas you can eat the same thing and have no negative reaction whatsoever. And it is still too early to tell just how influential estrogen's role is in these situations overall. But my clinical and research experiences do suggest that dips in estrogen levels are a factor in angioneurotic edema.

RELIEVING ALLERGIC EDEMA. The simplest and most common way to relieve allergic edema is with antihistamines or cortisone, an antiinflammatory agent. In the future, we may be able to treat a tendency toward allergic edema with estrogen supplement therapy, but we need to obtain much more information before we know for certain that this treatment approach is viable.

PULMONARY PROBLEMS

If you're having some trouble breathing deeply, or if you're coughing a lot or are very hoarse—and you're sure it's not caused by a simple cold or a bout with the flu—you may have a pulmonary problem. Don't worry; such problems are rarely dangerous and certainly common. Many transitional women encounter changes involving their lungs, trachea, bronchi, and other breathing apparatus.

Sometimes women report changes for the better. For instance, if you've spent years suffering with asthma, you may find that your symptoms may start leveling off somewhat as you move into your forties. However, some transitional women find they suffer from heightened attacks of hay fever. The most serious problem by far is lung cancer, for which you are at greater risk the older you get.

We're not sure why certain pulmonary ailments seem to intensify after age thirty-five. It's possible that a decline in sex hormones may play a role. Decreasing levels of estrogen, for instance, might indirectly affect the pulmonary system by reducing certain lung lipid substances that lubricate and thus ease the movement of the lungs. At this time, however, estrogen's impact is only speculation.

It's likely that the cumulative effect of several other factors that affect the lungs may begin to show up during the transitional years. Over the course of your lifetime, your lungs have been affected by smoking, hazardous work conditions (in chemical labs, health labs, knitting mills, and so on), activities that make you hyperventilate (such as childbirth), allergic reactions, and inhaled contaminants. It's likely that each one had only a subtle influence upon your health at the time. Their cumulative effect, however, may cause the problems that begin to appear in the transitional years, ranging from fairly benign breathing difficulties such as coughing attacks, hay fever, and sinusitis to such serious illnesses as lung cancer.

How to breathe easier.

Treatments for pulmonary problems vary widely with the condition, but they all share one goal: easing your ability to breathe. Space doesn't permit me to go into each specific problem and treatment method, but perhaps it is enough to say that even if you suffer from such problems, you needn't worry. In most cases, they can be managed, if not completely cured.

Hay fever sufferers or asthmatics can get great relief with the new inhalers—Brethaire or Bronkometer—which contain medications that open up the bronchi. If you have an allergic problem, antihistamines and steroids can help. If your doctor knows precisely what you're allergic to, "allergy shots" can be very effective (although not for food allergies). Today even lung cancer, when caught early, can be treated successfully.

GYNECOLOGICAL CANCERS

I hesitated to include cancer in this book because it is not a disease for which transitional women are at unusually high risk. Since millions of women in this age group are afflicted, however, I would not have felt right about excluding it, either. Besides, there's lots of good news concerning cancer these days. A diagnosis of cancer is by no means the death sentence it was in the past. When detected early, many cancers can either be cured or so well managed that patients can live a full, productive life.

Still and all, getting a cancer diagnosis can be a mind-numbing experience. Initially, at least, cancer patients feel their lives are totally out of control, and the emotional wallop reverberates throughout their network of family and friends. But with time and treatment, cancer patients and their families adjust, and may find that after treatment is completed, life goes on much as it did before diagnosis.

Prevention and early detection have a great deal to do with cancer success stories. I urge you to learn how to cut your risk and to be checked regularly enough to insure that if a problem does develop, it's detected early.

Breast cancer.

Menopausal women are most at risk for breast cancer, but many transitional women also find themselves facing this disease. In fact, breast cancer is the most common form of malignancy in women aged thirty-five to fifty. The risk is particularly high if you have a first-degree relative—such as a mother or sister—who already has (or had) the disease. The risk goes up even more if that relative was premenopausal at the time she developed cancer or if the cancer was in both breasts. Other factors that appear to be associated with breast cancer but over which you have little or no control are:

- *Early menstruation, before age eleven.*
- *Late menopause (after fifty).*
- *Giving birth for the first time after age thirty or not at all.*

Some physicians believe that fybrocystic disease (FCD) is a precursor to cancer, but new evidence suggests that that's not true and that women with the benign breast lumps characteristic of FCD are at no greater risk for breast cancer than women without FCD. (For a more complete discussion of FCD, see Chapter Eight.)

Many women worry that estrogen therapy or birth control pills may increase their likelihood of developing breast cancer. It is true that estrogen can play a role in the spread of cancer once it has developed. Specifically, women who have estrogen-dependent breast tumors should not take estrogen because the hormone could stimulate tumor cells to spread to other parts of the body and grow.

But for women who do not have estrogen-dependent tumors and are not at high risk for breast cancer, there isn't any clear evidence to suggest that low levels of estrogen used in estrogen therapy or found in birth control pills should be dangerous. As I mentioned on page 61, a 1992 review of major studies on estrogen, BCP, and breast cancer concluded that neither BCP nor estrogen has been clearly associated with greater risk for breast cancer. There are exceptions, however, and these involve a slight increase of breast cancer in women who have taken BCP or estrogen in high doses for many, many years. Still, the case for or against estrogen varies with each individual, so be sure to discuss thoroughly all the pros and cons with your doctor.

REDUCING YOUR RISK OF BREAST CANCER. Cancer experts point to a few things you can do to try to reduce your risk of developing the disease.

• *Cut your fat intake to 30 percent or less of your total calories.* Replacing much of the fatty meat and higher fat dairy products in your diet with more high-fiber fruits, vegetables, and whole grains will help reduce fat intake and help rid the body of toxins as well.
• *Increase your intake of vitamin C,* an antioxidant that seems to fight cancer-causing agents in your body.
• *Stop smoking.*
• *Limit alcohol intake to moderate amounts;* that is, no more than two drinks per day.
• *Increase the amount of omega-3 acids in your diet.* These are the fatty acids found in such fish as salmon, anchovies, herring, sardines, trout, and shad. The reason: a major study by Dr. Rashida Karmali, published in 1989 in the *Journal of the National Cancer Institute,* showed diets

high in omega-3s decreased incidence and growth of tumors, particularly breast and prostate tumors.
- *Wear a lead collar and apron if you have any dental X-rays taken* in order to avoid any unnecessary radiation.

For a while, some women who were at *very* high risk for breast cancer were choosing to undergo prophylactic mastectomies, the removal of healthy breasts to eliminate the chance for breast cancer. Today, this procedure is usually reserved for patients with cancer in one breast—the other, healthy breast is removed as a precaution. Clearly, however, prophylactic mastectomy is a radical alternative and deserves much personal consideration and a great deal of discussion between you and your doctor before you have it done.

DETECTING BREAST CANCER. Your best chance for beating most breast cancer is to have it diagnosed early, before the malignancy has a chance to spread any further. Examine your breasts each month, sometime during the two weeks after your period, when there's the least amount of lumpiness or swelling. Additionally, your gynecologist should examine your breasts every six months, or at least yearly if you're under forty.

For years now, the American Cancer Society has recommended that you get routine mammograms: once between ages thirty-five and forty; every eighteen to twenty-four months in your forties; and yearly after age fifty. However, some new research has suggested that women under fifty don't benefit from mammography. Specifically, Canadian and Swedish studies could not demonstrate that women in this age group who get mammography have a better survival rate from cancer than women who do not undergo this test. They did, however, see a marked survival advantage for women fifty and over.

One of the main reasons that mammograms may not always reveal a lump in the breasts of transitional women is that their breasts are too dense to allow a clear picture. So even with mammography, many malignancies go undetected.

As a result of this new information, controversy has erupted on when and how often women under fifty should get a mammogram. The National Cancer Institute has recently issued new guidelines that recommend yearly mammograms only for women fifty and over; the organization leaves it up to individual doctors and their patients to decide what to do before age fifty. The American Cancer Society, however, is sticking to its old guidelines.

As for me, I believe that since today's mammograms use a very low dose of radiation, so that there is no real risk, the potential benefits of detecting cancer in its earliest stages far outweigh the downside. My recommendation for a transitional woman is that if you are examined regularly by your doctor and are not at high risk, you should have an initial mammogram at age forty, then another every two years between the ages of forty and fifty. After age fifty, of course, I recommend annual mammograms.

Please make sure you have your tests done at reputable diagnostic centers. Some women have insurance policies that dictate where they can go for mammograms, and too often these are not the best places available. If you can possibly swing it financially, I would strongly urge you to go somewhere your doctor recommends highly. Going to a first-rate facility with excellent technicians and the most up-to-date equipment will increase your chances for a reliable mammogram and a good interpretation of the film. This will help you detect any malignancies as early as possible.

Remember: even if you do find a lump, it doesn't mean you have cancer. Even so, you must have it checked and, if necessary, biopsied immediately, since a biopsy is the only surefire way to confirm a diagnosis. (For more information on breast biopsies, see Chapter Eight.)

TREATING BREAST CANCER. If by some chance a malignancy is discovered in your breast, treatment will depend on the pathology of the cancer—that is, the type of cells the cancer involves and how they behave microscopically. But options generally include:

- *Excisional biopsy.* This is the removal of a small tumor (less than one half inch in diameter) during the diagnostic biopsy.
- *Lumpectomy.* This procedure involves the removal of the entire mass along with normal tissue all around the cancer.
- *Simple mastectomy.* More extensive than a lumpectomy, a mastectomy calls for the removal of all breast tissue, but the surrounding muscle and tissue are left intact.
- *Radical mastectomy.* This approach, more accurately called a *modified radical mastectomy*, includes the removal of the breast as well as some of the surrounding arm muscle; the procedure is always modified to fit the needs of the particular patient.

(NOTE: In all cases, the nodes under your arm will be checked to see if the cancer has spread to them also.)

After surgery, most breast cancer patients undergo radiation and/or chemotherapy. The length and aggressiveness of this treatment again depend on the pathology and "stage" of the cancer; most cancers have five stages, stage 0 (also called *carcinoma in situ*, or CIS) being least extensive and stage 4 the most. Approximately 85 percent of breast cancers discovered in transitional women are at stage 1. An anti-estrogen medication such as tamoxifen citrate may also be part of the follow-up treatment.

Right now the National Cancer Institute is funding some potentially exciting research to see if tamoxifen can actually *prevent* breast cancer. In clinical trials that will eventually involve some 16,000 women at high risk for breast cancer, women are being given tamoxifen prophylactically. Because the study is a long-term one, results are several years away.

Cervical cancer.

If cervical cancer is found early, it has better than a 90 percent cure rate. The best way to catch precancerous conditions—which can be detected up to two years before an actual malignancy exists—as well as early malignancies is by means of a Pap smear. Every transitional woman should have this simple test done at least once, and preferably twice, a year.

If the results of your Pap test are not normal, this does not necessarily signal cancer. Sometimes, the abnormality is caused by dysplasia, atypical changes in cervical tissue. If dysplasia is mild, your doctor will probably not attempt to treat it but will continue to observe it closely. If it's moderate, he or she may want to do a colposcopy, an office procedure in which your doctor looks at the outside and inside of the cervix with a microscope. If the problem looks suspicious, your physician may take a biopsy to rule out cancer.

If there's no malignancy, the dysplasia can be effectively treated with cryosurgery (freezing the cervix), cautery, laser, or electrocauterization (via a Loop Electrode Excision Procedure, a.k.a. LEEP) of the cervix. Once the area heals, fresh, normal tissue will usually appear and the dysplasia will be eliminated.

TREATING CERVICAL CANCER. If a malignancy exists, treatment depends on the stage of the cancer. A stage 0 cancer is the least malignant; the diseased tissue can often be removed by a cone biopsy (scooping out the malignant tissue) of the cervix. If the cancer is advanced, a hysterectomy may be required. Surgery may or may not be followed by radiation and/or chemotherapy.

REDUCING YOUR RISK OF CERVICAL CANCER. As I mentioned earlier, there appears to be a connection between diet and cancer, so eat as healthfully as you can. Some researchers believe eating foods rich in the antioxidant vitamin C is a good idea since it appears to help protect your body against the damaging effects of free radicals and, thus, to help ward off cancer. (For more information on antioxidants, as well as recommendations for a healthful diet, see Chapter Two.) STDs and cigarette smoke have been linked to cervical cancer, so avoid both.

Uterine cancer.

If found early, uterine cancer has a 95 percent cure rate! It helps that there are some common warning signs—specifically, mid-cycle bleeding or irregular bleeding before or after the menstrual cycle. The best way to confirm a diagnosis of cancer of the uterus, also known as endometrial cancer, is through endometrial sampling. This is a simple and relatively painless office procedure in which tissue is removed from the uterine lining and then analyzed. If your doctor finds anything suspicious, he or she would next perform a fractional D&C to confirm or disprove any malignancy.

TREATING UTERINE CANCER. Surgery is the first line of treatment for uterine cancer. Usually, patients will undergo a total hysterectomy in which the surgeon removes not only the cervix and uterus but also both fallopian tubes and both ovaries in order to prevent the cancer from spreading to those organs. (Removing the ovaries also helps reduce the estrogen levels.) Depending on the stage of malignancy and how aggressive the particular cancer is, the patient would probably undergo some course of radiation before or after surgery. After surgery, she may also have chemotherapy to reduce and, it is hoped, eliminate any chance that the cancer will spread.

REDUCING YOUR RISK OF UTERINE CANCER. Researchers believe that a few tactics may help you cut your risk for uterine cancer. First, keep your weight at the levels suggested in the weight chart on page 38. Obesity—that is, being more than 20 percent above recommended weight levels—has been linked with uterine cancer. Second, if you are a good candidate for them, take birth control pills. Research has shown that women who take birth control pills are at lower risk of uterine cancer.
More good ideas:

• *Avoid and/or treat hypertension,* a condition that has been associated with uterine cancer.

• *Keep diabetes under control.* Women with untreated diabetes are at greater risk of uterine cancer, although we're not exactly sure why. It may be that higher risk is related to the obesity of some diabetic women, particularly those whose diabetes is out of control, than the disease itself.

• *Treat menstrual problems*—whatever their cause—since women with irregular periods have a higher chance for uterine cancer. (See Chapter Three for an in-depth discussion of menstrual problems.)

Ovarian cancer.

I can't blame anyone for being frightened of ovarian cancer. Although it's far less common than breast cancer—only about one in eighty women develops the disease, as opposed to breast cancer's one-in-nine statistic—it can be more destructive because it is rarely detected in its early stages. The reason ovarian cancer goes undetected is that it usually causes no symptoms, at least initially. By the time symptoms appear and the disease is detected, the cancer has usually spread beyond the ovaries to other organs.

REDUCING YOUR RISK FOR OVARIAN CANCER. If for any reason you have to have a hysterectomy, your doctor may advise you to have your ovaries removed at the same time to insure you'll never get ovarian cancer. At many medical centers, women over thirty-five who need hysterectomies are routinely given the option of having their ovaries removed (a procedure called *oophorectomy*.)

This is okay for women over forty-five, particularly if they have a strong family history of ovarian cancer (a close relative—a mother, sister, maternal aunt, or grandmother with the disease), have already gone through menopause, or are very close to it. Otherwise, I'd advise transitional women against having their ovaries removed for several reasons.

- *Your estrogen levels are already beginning to drop.* Losing your ovaries will make those levels plummet and send you into menopause prematurely and immediately.
- *Not all women can take estrogen replacement therapy after having their ovaries removed.* For some women ERT causes too much gastrointestinal upset or allergic side effects. If you can't take estrogen after surgery, you'll have

little protection against menopausal symptoms and estrogen-deficiency diseases.

- *Your ovaries probably have a lifelong protective function.* Even after menopause, they don't shrivel up and die. For one thing, they make a hormone called *androstenedione*, which some feel may be important in maintaining your sex drive and preventing osteoporosis.
- *Removing healthy ovaries offers few benefits compared with the risks.* It has been estimated that doctors have to do 700 oophorectomies to prevent one case of ovarian cancer! We have to ask, How many of the remaining 699 women suffer long-term complications from the loss of the ovaries or from the surgery itself?

If you must have an ovary removed (for example, to treat ovarian cysts, tubovarian infection, or such benign tumors as dermoids), ask your doctor to leave intact as much healthy tissue as practical so as to minimize your risk for estrogen deficiency.

Several less drastic measures can help you cut your risk for ovarian cancer.

- *Consider taking birth control pills.* If you are a good candidate for them, oral contraceptives reduce the risk of ovarian cancer. As I explained in Chapter Five, many women over thirty-five can safely use this form of birth control.
- *Avoid talcum powder.* Don't dust talcum powder on your panties or in your vaginal area. A 1992 Harvard study showed that women who used talcum powder on their genital area daily over the course of several years were at greater risk for ovarian cancer than women who did not. If you want to use a powder, choose one with cornstarch instead.
- *Limit the amount of dairy products you eat.* Some studies suggest that eating excessive amounts (more than

four servings a day) of such products as yogurt and milk could increase your risk of ovarian cancer and early menopause.

• *Have a thorough gynecological checkup at least once a year.* Your gynecologist is the most likely person to detect ovarian cancer at an early stage, when it can be treated successfully.

DETECTING OVARIAN CANCER. One diagnostic technique is a simple blood test called a CA-125. CA-125 is an antigen that may be shed into the blood by ovarian cancer cells. Elevated levels of this antigen are found in 80 percent of women with ovarian cancer, which is why doctors often use the CA-125 to screen for ovarian malignancies. However, the test is not sensitive or specific enough to *diagnose* cancer; sometimes, women with benign conditions will have an elevated CA-125.

If the results of your CA-125 look suspicious *or* if your doctor suspects a problem during your checkup—for instance, if he or she feels any enlargement of the ovary that's not related to menstrual cycles—a transvaginal ultrasound may be performed. In this test, sound waves are beamed through the vagina at the ovaries. As with any ultrasound procedure, these reflected waves are picked up and transformed into pictures of the ovaries that can be viewed on a television screen and on a printout.

If your doctor is still concerned about malignancy, he or she will probably perform a laparoscopy (described in Chapter Six) or a laparotomy, the surgical opening of the abdomen, so that the suspicious tissue may be biopsied and the presence of ovarian cancer confirmed or ruled out.

Cancer Treatment After Thirty-five

I hope you'll never need the advice I'm going to offer here. But I want you to have it, just in case. It concerns the link between early menopause and cancer treatment.

Thirty-six-year-old Celeste was terrified when a biopsy of a skin blemish revealed a malignant melanoma. Luckily it was detected very early on, and after Celeste received several months of radiation and chemotherapy, the disease went into remission. Celeste's prognosis was excellent.

Yet after her treatment, Celeste, the mother of a four-year-old daughter, came to see me quite concerned. Her periods had not returned. "Bernie, my husband and I really want to have another baby. Will that ever be possible?" I told Celeste the truth: there was a chance that she might go into early menopause because of radiation damage to the ovaries that might have occurred during treatment. But there was also a chance that her cycles might resume. All we could do was wait and see.

Celeste's husband was transferred to a new division of his company and the family moved. About three months later, I got a note from her saying her periods had resumed. Six months after that, another note: Celeste was pregnant!

Unfortunately, not every woman is so lucky. While in most women the side effects of cancer therapy are temporary and the ovaries recover in time, some do go through menopause because of side effects from chemotherapy or radiation therapy. (Obviously, surgical removal of the reproductive organs results in immediate menopause.)

So what can you do about it? If cancer is discovered, speak up and ask your doctor if your ovaries are in harm's way. If they are, ask if anything can be done to protect them. Your doctor may be able to change the mix of chemotherapy drugs to prevent ovarian damage without compromising the treatment's effectiveness in any way.

If your ovaries can't be protected, going on estrogen therapy after cancer treatment might help. This is not an option, however, if your cancer is estrogen-dependent. In fact, if you have an estrogen-dependent cancer, treatment that shuts down your ovaries—and, thus, your estrogen production—is a good idea. But even then, there's an option open for women who desire children in the future: you can donate your eggs before treatment for in vitro fertilization. These eggs can be frozen and then, at a later date, after your cancer treatment is over, thawed and fertilized in a test tube and implanted in your uterus (assuming it was not removed in surgery) or in the uterus of a surrogate. Even without your ovaries, you may still be able to have your own child. (For more information on alternative ways to have a baby, see Chapter Six.)

No one wants to consider the possibility of a serious illness. With luck, you'll never have to confront one, but even if you do, there's always hope. New diagnostic procedures and state-of-the-art treatments have dramatically improved the likelihood that you'll recover completely. As long as you know what to expect—the downsides and risks as well as the best, most effective treatments—and as long as you're willing to become an active partner with your doctors, you're more likely to beat whatever disease you face.

11

A Doctor's Guide to Looking Good

> - How to Have Younger-Looking Skin
> - Controlling Adult Acne
> - Improving the Appearance of Your Hair
> - Dealing with Unwanted Hair
> - Troublesome Veins
> - Protecting Your Smile

Because I'm a physician, making sure you *feel* good has been much more important to me than making sure you *look* good. But over the years I've learned that the two are not always so separate. Your appearance—how healthy your skin looks, how shiny your hair, how bright your smile—is often a good indicator of what's happening beneath the surface.

I always look carefully at my patients' outer selves for signs of any health problems. Certain changes may be subtle but meaningful. Unusually rough, dry skin, for instance, can indicate an underactive thyroid; yellowed eyes can signal jaundice; and bright red palms may be a sign of liver disease.

Of course, there are other subtle changes in your appearance that don't mean anything's wrong. Those first few wrinkles, strands of gray hair, and slightly droopier breasts are the perfectly normal results of the natural aging process, the gradual slowdown of cell activity and steadily shifting hormones. If we lived in another culture—one that did not idolize youth the way we do here in the United States—you might wear those changes proudly as badges of life experience. In that case, this chapter would not be necessary. Through our Western eyes, however, the physical changes you're experiencing can damage your overall sense of well-being.

Some transitional women manage to revel in their new, more mature looks, but the vast majority feel a tug of anxiety when they begin to notice a less youthful face and body reflected back at them. That's where this chapter comes in.

I want transitional women to feel their best. And in our society, feeling your best means looking your best. So let's take an honest look at your appearance, understand what's behind the changes you've noticed, and explore what you can—and can't—do to keep yourself looking as good as or even better than you ever have before.

How to Have Younger-Looking Skin

Not only is the skin your body's largest organ, it's also the one that most ruthlessly reveals your age. Just compare your skin to the way it was when you were twenty; it's undoubtedly drier, less taut, more lined, or wrinkled today. Some of that has to do with years of exposure to the elements, particularly sun, cold, and wind, but most of these changes must be blamed on a biological process called *atrophism*.

Atrophism is the wasting away or shrinking of tissue. It's caused by a lack of cell activity at a particular site. As you age, your cells become "lazier"; they don't grow and develop as fast as they once did. Thus, your body tissues gradually begin to:

- *Regenerate more slowly.*
- *Take longer to heal.*
- *Lose some of their subcutaneous lipids* (the fat beneath the skin).
- *Actively break down and degenerate.*

Atrophism of the skin begins slowly and subtly when you're in your early twenties. At about age thirty-six, the very start of your transitional years, it speeds up and its symptoms become more noticeable. Specifically, as the production of new cells slows, several things happen:

- *Your skin's outer layer, the epidermis, can't regenerate as quickly,* so your skin begins to look more dull.
- *Supporting fibers in the dermis, the skin's middle layer, break down and lose elasticity,* so your skin starts to sag and wrinkles begin to appear.
- *The fatty tissue below the dermis begins to break down,* which can change the angles and contours of your face.
- *The oil and sweat glands in your skin become less effective,* which leads to drier skin that can begin to crack and occasionally peel.
- *Your skin may break out more.*

When you're young, your skin rejuvenates itself every thirty days in a rather straightforward process: new tissue is manufactured at the base of the epidermis and, during the days that follow, makes its way up to the surface, where eventually it's sloughed off. As you get older, this process slows. The skin you see—the outermost tissue of your epidermis, called the *stratum corneum*—is literally "older"; with age, more dead skin cells accumulate before they are sloughed off and replaced. Other factors that conspire to age your skin include a diminished blood supply to the skin, breakage of elastic fibers, and a decrease in the amount of collagen. All of these factors are exacerbated by declining estrogen levels, which, as we've already discussed in an earlier chapter, further dries out the skin. The result: duller-looking, less "youthful" skin.

While you may never be able to recapture the "glow" of youth, you can come a lot closer by following these tips:

- *Use an exfoliant.* Ever wonder why most men's skin seems to look better than women's? In large part, it has to do with shaving. By shaving every day, men scrape off their stratum corneum, the outermost skin tissue, and help compensate for the slowdown in the rejuvenating cycle.

You can do the same by using a gentle exfoliant or facial scrub on your skin. Talk to your dermatologist or just visit a beauty aids store to discover the best one for you. Be careful not to scrub too hard or too often, though; excessive pressure can damage your skin.

- *Drink six to eight glasses of water a day.* Remember, you can't replace moisture from the outside in, but only from the inside out.
- *Make sure your diet is rich in vitamin A,* which promotes healthier skin. You'll find it in dark, leafy greens and in yellow and orange vegetables and fruits. Vitamin C is also important since it keeps your capillaries healthier, allowing oxygen to reach your skin tissues. Good sources include citrus fruits, cantaloupe, broccoli, and tomatoes.

- *Protect your skin from the cold and wind* by using moisturizers when you go out and by covering as much of your skin as possible. In cold, dry weather, use a humidifier indoors.
- *Use gentle soaps when bathing or showering,* then pat your skin dry.
- *Apply an emollient,* such as an oil-based moisturizing cream, after bathing, when your skin is still damp, in order to seal in moisture.

Minimizing wrinkles and sags.

Gently pinch the back of your hand so that you lift the skin up a bit. Now pay close attention to how long it takes for your skin to return to its previous position. A few seconds, right? Well, if you'd done this test when you were in your teens or early twenties, it wouldn't have taken nearly that long; instead, your skin would have sprung back into shape almost immediately.

The reason it takes longer now is that your skin has lost some of its elasticity. Your dermis, the inner layer of the skin, has shrunk a bit. Valiantly, your epidermis tries to cover it, but it's become too loose to do so evenly. Furthermore, as you age, you lose collagen, the fibrous protein that helps keep skin taut. As collagen levels drop, your skin begins to lose its shape. The result: those first few wrinkles that usually appear initially as creases at the corners of your eyes, lines in your forehead and between your eyebrows, and in the deeper lines that run from the sides of your nose down to the corners of your mouth.

Wrinkling is inevitable. But how fast you'll wrinkle and to what extent depends on a few factors, some of which you can control and some of which you cannot.

- *Heredity.* Wrinkling tends to run in the family. If your mother wrinkled early and deeply, chances are you will, too. Taking good care of your skin, however, can help offset this particular genetic tendency.
- *Environment.* If you've had too much exposure to sun, cold, and wind, and haven't done much about protecting your skin, you've probably aged your skin prematurely. This means you may wrinkle earlier and more extensively than you might like. You can't undo what has been done, but you can be more careful, starting today.
- *Smoking.* Chalk up another black mark against smoking. When you puff away, you actually reduce the size of your blood vessels. Decreasing blood flow to the skin prevents sufficient oxygen from reaching the cells and thus encourages wrinkling.
- *Your personality.* If you're a very expressive, emotive person, you probably have a constantly changing array of facial expressions. Some experts feel that this continuous stretching of the skin on your face can promote wrinkles, although I wouldn't advise anybody to tone down her personality in order to spare herself a wrinkle or two!
- *Pressure on the skin.* If you put continuous pressure on one area of the skin for hours at a time—say, you always sleep with one side of your face resting on the pillow—you'll tend to get more wrinkling on that side of your face. The best sleeping position to slow the wrinkling process is on your back.

As I said before, everyone gets wrinkles. *Everyone.* But you can adopt a few strategies that will help keep yours to a minimum.

- *Avoid the sun.* I know you've heard this a million times, so make this a million and one. I would be remiss if I didn't point out that exposure to the sun's damaging ultraviolet rays undeniably promotes wrinkling (not to mention skin cancer). Just take a look at those women (and men) who seem to have a constant deep, dark tan. Up close, their skin looks like old, cracked leather.

Whenever possible, avoid prolonged exposure to the sun. When you spend time outside, protect your skin by using a sunscreen with a minimum sun protection factor (SPF) of 15 to 30. If your skin is very fair, move up to an SPF of 45 to 50.

- *Use skin products containing alphahydroxy acids (AHAs).* For years, cosmetics companies have done a hard sell on lotions and creams, overemphasizing their ability to reduce wrinkles, moisturize skin, and even eliminate age spots. Most didn't do any such thing. But now dermatologists have hit upon something that may really work: alphahydroxy acids (or AHAs), naturally occurring substances found in such fruits as grapes, apples, and citrus, and in other products such as sour milk. Products with AHAs such as lactic acid and glycolic acid apparently increase the number of glycosaminoglycans, the spongy water-holding molecules in the middle layer of your skin. This makes your skin more hydrated and, therefore, more glowing and less wrinkly.

It's still too soon to gauge just how much AHA is needed to work effectively. An over-the-counter skin preparation may contain no more than 15 percent AHA; products containing 20 to 25 percent or more AHA require a prescription. It's also too soon to tell how long the results may last. Still, the future of AHA-enhanced products looks promising.

- *Try Retin-A.* If you find your wrinkles very upsetting, your dermatologist might prescribe Retin-A (tretinoin), a medication related to vitamin A that does seem to slow the wrinkling process. Retin-A is available in a cream, gel, or liquid and is applied directly to the skin. But be patient: it can take several months before you see any improvement. Do not try to speed up the process by using more than the prescribed amount; if you use too much, your skin can overdose and become extremely sun-sensitive, itchy, painful, scaly, or red and mottled. Be sure to follow your doctor's directions carefully. Also, Retin-A should not be used by pregnant women since no well-controlled studies have been done to gauge its effect on the fetus.

- *Collagen injections.* Injecting a form of collagen (mixed with your own blood serum) directly into crease lines almost immediately makes those wrinkles fade. Results last anywhere from about nine months to two years. But be forewarned: some people are allergic to collagen. Your doctor should do a sensitivity test to assess your body's reaction *before* starting treatment. Another possible drawback: collagen treatments can be very expensive.

- *Dermabrasion.* Skin peeling—using chemicals such as phenol derivatives to burn away old, wrinkled, or scarred skin so that the amount of collagen increases and new, smoother skin can be revealed—can give you a more youthful look. Dermabrasion can also be done mechanically; the doctor uses a skin-planing tool to sand down the wrinkled areas.

Dermabrasion does not come with a guarantee, however. In some people, when new epidermal layers grow back to replace the ones that have been peeled away, the skin can look shiny, pink, unpigmented, or uneven. It's hard to anticipate the results since every individual's skin heals differently. Your best insurance is to go to a professional who is highly experienced and skilled in this technique.

- *Cosmetic surgery.* More and more transitional women are opting for the most extreme solution to their wrinkling and sagging: surgery. Face-lifts eliminate skin folds and, if done well, make you look more rested and years younger. Eyelid tucks reduce drooping eyelids and bags around the eyes. The results of both procedures last anywhere from three to seven years before you may need to repeat them.

No surgery, particularly cosmetic surgery, should be taken lightly. First, none of the techniques are permanent. Second, if general anesthesia is involved, you run the risks inherent in any major operation. Additionally, while prices are becoming more affordable, these procedures are still expensive. And if you're not happy with the results, there's not much you can do about it except go through more surgery—and the outcome is never guaranteed.

Controlling Adult Acne

Maybe you were one of those lucky teens who wasn't plagued by acne. So why now, at age forty, do you find you're breaking out on your chin, jawline, neck, chest, and back, particularly around the time of your period?

During the transitional years, your skin is very sensitive to hormonal shifts that take place each month. There are two types of skin pores: sebaceous glands and follicles. Normally, your sebaceous glands shed dead cells and release excess oil. During menstruation, however, these pores close up in response to hormonal changes. Dead cells clog the pores, oil builds up, and bacteria multiply, resulting in what we know as whiteheads and blackheads on your face, chest, and back.

Pimples also erupt, but they're not the kind you're used to: these are raised, firm, sometimes uncomfortable but rarely pussy cysts. Applying warm compresses will not bring them to a head, and no matter what creams and salves you use on them, they tend to hang around. The reason: these cysts are caused by sebaceous glands responding to changes in estrogen and progesterone—and topical acne preparations and compresses do nothing to change your hormonal mix.

Other causes of adult acne.

Hormonal shifts aren't the only factors that lead to adult acne. Others include:

- *Stress.* We have no irrefutable evidence linking stress with acne, but many women have noticed a connection. It makes sense: under stress, your adrenal glands do pump out a lot more androgen, which may promote these eruptions.
- *Too much makeup, not enough cleansing.* Heavy makeup can clog your pores, which is why some dermatologists recommend using a light moisturizer under your makeup as a protective barrier. At the end of each day you should also make sure you remove all traces of makeup with a mild cleanser so that your pores can "breathe."
- *Touching.* When you rest your hand on your face or hold the phone against your chin, the resulting physical pressure—not to mention the grime and grit—seems to aggravate acne. If you pop or pick at pimples, you can inflame the area, enlarge the eruption, and increase scarring.
- *Drugs.* Certain drugs seem to promote breakouts. These include danazol (for endometriosis), lithium (for a mood disorder), iodides (for thyroid problems), and anabolic steroids (used to pump up muscles).

Remedies.

Unfortunately, I know of no miracle remedies for adult acne. But you can try a few options:

- *Over-the-counter (OTC) treatments.* Topical OTC preparations with benzoyl peroxide or salicylic acid can accelerate the rate at which dead cells are sloughed off. OTC medications containing sulfur and resorcinol can dry up blemishes, but they're often too drying for transitional women's skin.
- *Prescription drugs.* I've already mentioned Retin-A (see page 269). This medication helps to accelerate the turnover of skin cells and prevents clogged pores.

If your acne is severe, your doctor might prescribe isotretinoin, which you may recognize by its trade name, Acutane. Like Retin-A, Acutane is also derived from vitamin A—but don't let that fool you. It has a different chemical makeup from Retin-A and is a more powerful drug. Whereas Retin-A is applied topically to the skin, Acutane is taken orally and can have severe side effects; it can cause inflammatory bowel disease and liver problems. It should never be taken by anyone who knows or even suspects she is pregnant, because Acutane has been strongly linked to birth defects. Another negative: Acutane raises cholesterol and triglycerides, so if your doctor prescribes it, make sure you have your cholesterol checked regularly.

- *Eat a balanced diet.* Contrary to what your mother may have told you, neither chocolate nor fried foods cause acne, although diets high in fat can increase sebum, the fatty secretion of the sebaceous glands, which can lead to greater skin problems. It goes almost without saying, however, that eating a well-balanced diet rich in fruits, vegetables, whole grains, and complex carbohydrates—and drinking six to eight eight-ounce glasses of water each day—will give you the best shot at clear, healthy skin.

Improving the Appearance of Your Hair

You may have noticed that your hair is thinner, drier, more brittle, and less shiny than it used to be. Well, there are several reasons for that. One is that your hair is made up of a number of "plates" (thin, flat segments, the main ingredient of which is keratin) that come together and make it strong. As you get older, the number of plates in each growing hair gradually declines, and the plates don't adhere as well, making hair more brittle and prone to split ends.

You will not be surprised to hear that hormones play a role. When you're young, the androgen in your body promotes hair growth; estrogen makes hair lustrous. In your transitional years, androgen levels increase, but this causes you to *lose* rather than grow hair. Moreover, as estrogen begins to decrease at this point in your life, the glands in and around your scalp secrete less oil, which makes your hair drier and more dull. For women whose hair has always been too oily, this is good news. They still have enough natural lubrication to keep their hair shiny. But for many women, drier hair means less manageable and less attractive hair.

Finally, drier, more brittle hair may also have something to do with the cumulative effect of years of coloring, straightening, curling, and blow-drying your hair. Like it or not, all that processing may be beginning to catch up to you.

What can you do to reverse this process and improve the health and appearance of your hair? I'm far from a hair pundit, but the experts I've spoken with recommend these few tips:

- *Try using hair products that contain vitamin A and biotin.* These substances play an important role in keratin formation and in keeping your hair's "plates" tight.
- *Use a mild shampoo that won't overdry your hair.*
- *Don't wash your hair too often.*
- *Dry it carefully.* Ideally, you should let your hair dry at least partially on its own; then, when you use your dryer, keep the source of the heated air at least six to eight inches away from your head. If you towel-dry, don't scrub; that can damage the hair.
- *Avoid harsh chemicals.* Hair colors or other treatments that contain peroxide or ammonia can dry your hair out even more.

Your hair may be turning gray faster than you'd like, but gray hair is a fact of life. As you get older, the pigment-producing cells at the base of your hair roots start slowing down, and as they do, your hair becomes more and more gray. These gray hairs are more coarse and brittle than those with color.

I happen to like gray hair—and I'm most grateful that I still have a respectable amount on my own head! But if you really hate your gray—and I admit it does make most people look older—find a good colorist and go to it! I recommend you get expert help from someone who understands hair and hair products. Perming and coloring can be a disastrous mix if you're not careful.

Whatever product you select, be sure to test it on a tiny patch of skin first to make sure you're not allergic to it. You should actually do *two* patch tests: an initial one, then another two days later. Be aware that you can also develop an allergy to a product you've used safely for years. If you notice any hives, swelling around the eyes, and/or severe itching, particularly around the scalp, do another test before continuing, no matter how long you've been using the product.

Dealing with Unwanted Hair

Because your estrogen levels are gradually declining, the male hormones in your bloodstream are no longer fully counterbalanced by female hormones. Result: you may notice the growth of unwanted facial hairs, particularly on your chin and upper lip. You may also notice more hair growth around your nipples and from your navel to your pubic area.

Since this hair is in no way harmful, you don't need to do anything about it. And if you're undergoing estrogen therapy for any one of a number of conditions we've already discussed in earlier chapters, the estrogen will alleviate the problem. If you're not on estrogen and the excess hair is making you feel less attractive, any one of these techniques might help:

- *Bleaching.* Using an over-the-counter bleaching preparation, even simple peroxide, can help camouflage unwanted hair. Just make sure you're not allergic to the bleach. (Once more, a simple patch test will tell the tale.)
- *Waxing.* It's a bit painful, but waxing helps pull hairs out by the roots, so you don't need to do it that often.
- *Tweezing.* Another way to pull hair out by the roots.
- *Depilatories.* You can buy any one of a number of chemical creams to rid yourself of hair. Some are more effective than others, but trial and error should lead you to a good one. Again, make sure you're not allergic.

- *Shaving.* It's the most basic way to remove hair, but it works. The biggest problem is the repetition: hair usually grows back within three or four days under most circumstances.
- *Electrolysis.* Using electric current to destroy hair follicles is an effective way to get rid of very coarse, actively growing hair. But when the hair being removed is caused by hormonal shifts, electrolysis is not a permanent solution and must be repeated every few weeks or months, depending on the individual. Still and all, it lasts a good deal longer than most hair-removal techniques.

Troublesome Veins

Among the most widespread complaints of transitional women are spider veins and varicose veins.

Spider veins.

Spider veins are those thin, broken, bluish, or reddish veins that appear just below your skin's surface. They're harmless, though many women find them unsightly. If they bother you, your dermatologist can get rid of them fairly easily through a process known as *sclerotherapy*. During this procedure, hypertonic saline (salt water) is injected into the veins, which floods them and turns them a less noticeable whitish color. Take note, however: this procedure can be quite costly and may not be covered by your insurance.

Varicose veins.

Varicose veins occur when certain small valves in the veins of the legs fail to function. Instead of flowing upward to the heart, blood pools in the veins, causing them to swell and appear as bulging, purplish lines. Although varicose veins can pose a real health threat on occasion, most women seek treatment for cosmetic rather than health reasons—which is why I decided to discuss them in this chapter. However, I don't want to minimize the importance of varicose veins, nor overlook the fact that they can be quite painful.

Certain factors can cause, or at least aggravate, varicose veins. Wearing overly tight clothing or sitting with your legs crossed for long periods of time restricts the flow of blood through the veins and promotes swelling. So can narrowing of the blood vessels caused by a buildup of lipids or fat on their inner walls. If you're very overweight and don't exercise regularly, you're also more likely to suffer a problem.

Varicose veins can increase your risk for blood clots. A small clot that occurs within these blood vessels can stop blood from flowing through them, resulting in a painful inflammation of the veins called thrombophlebitis. (See Chapter Ten for a more detailed discussion of thrombophlebitis.) It's possible for a clot to be thrown off to the lungs, the brain, or the heart, causing a serious medical problem.

Because there are no simple treatments for large, painful varicose veins, the best thing to do is to prevent them in the first place. If they run in your family, this may not be altogether possible. But you can minimize your risk for varicose veins by:

- *Exercising your legs* through such regular activities as walking, jogging, bicycling, hiking, and swimming.

- *Keeping your weight down* to recommended levels (see the weight chart on page 38).
- *Wearing elastic support stockings* when you're pregnant. Blood flow from the legs is slowed during pregnancy and the stockings help to encourage better flow.
- *Resting your legs* periodically and, at the same time, elevating them so that your feet are higher than your hips.
- *Avoiding sitting or standing for long periods of time.* Sitting with your legs crossed cuts off good circulation; standing encourages blood to pool in your legs.
- *Eating a high-fiber, low-fat diet* to promote cholesterol reduction and healthy circulation.

To alleviate the pain and discomfort of varicose veins that have already become problems, follow these suggestions:

- *Exercise.* Any gentle aerobic activity that helps veins pump blood back to the heart can help.
- *Wear support hose.* They will lend more elasticity to the connective tissue in your legs and therefore will help your blood circulate better.
- *Elevate your legs* above hip level several times every day.

If these options don't help, you may want to consider surgery. Unfortunately, sclerotherapy doesn't work on large, bulging varicose veins. Instead, bothersome veins are surgically removed by means of a procedure called "stripping." You should be aware, however, that other unsightly veins sometimes appear, so corrective surgery isn't something that should be done lightly.

Protecting Your Smile

In your transitional years, keeping your teeth looking white and bright is a bit harder now that you have to contend with years of coffee and tea stains. You might already be using some of those tooth-brightening toothpastes now on the market. A word of caution, though: some of those "brighteners" may be overly abrasive, so check with your dentist before making them part of your daily routine.

No amount of brushing will make your teeth as white as you'd probably like, and brushing does nothing for chipped or cracked teeth. If you want to improve your smile, consider cosmetic bonding. In a multistep procedure, a substance called composite (actually a plastic, glass, or quartz veneer that matches the color of your teeth) is applied to the tooth until the imperfection or stain is covered. Bonding can last for years, though at some point the procedure usually has to be repeated.

During the transitional years it's your gums, rather than your teeth, that need the lion's share of your time and attention. Periodontal disease is the biggest cause of tooth loss in the transitional years, so now's the time to focus on your gums. Here's why. As you grow older, bacteria that build up in your mouth—first in the form of *plaque*, a thin, colorless film that coats your teeth, and then as *tartar* or *calculus*, calcified plaque—can irritate your gums (gingiva), causing *gingivitis*, a superficial inflammation of your gums characterized by redness, swelling, and bleeding. If gingivitis is left untreated, the gum tissue around the base of the teeth can become damaged. Tiny pockets form that fill with bacteria-laden plaque. If still unchecked, the inflammation can develop into periodontitis, an advanced stage of gum disease in which the supporting tissues of the teeth are affected.

A Doctor's Guide to Looking Good

As you get older and your gums recede slightly, more of the root of each tooth is exposed to bacteria. As more root is exposed, the periodontal ligament may be destroyed and your tooth becomes loosened, then detached, from the gum. When the adjacent bone becomes affected, bone destruction will begin; if left untreated, in addition to tooth loss, the gum and bone under it will begin to break down.

The best way to protect your smile is to start paying careful attention to your gums now. Brushing and flossing twice a day help keep your teeth and gums relatively free of bacteria. Some dentists recommend using baking soda and peroxide instead of, or along with, fluoride toothpaste. Brushing and flossing also aid in massaging gums, which helps to prevent them from receding and in general keeps them healthier. Additionally, you need to see your dentist at least once a year, preferably twice, for a thorough, professional cleaning. Regular checkups and cleanings can help lower your risk for gingivitis or at least detect it at an early stage when it can be treated easily.

Looking your best goes hand in hand with attaining your peak level of health and vitality throughout your transitional years. Knowing you look great will help give you the confidence you need to move through the transitional years successfully and to help make the eventual move into menopause with self-assurance, grace, and vigor.

12

Finding Emotional Well-being

- Depression
- Anxiety and Panic Attacks
- Premenstrual Syndrome
- Understanding Blood Sugar
- Thyroid Problems
- Life Demands
- Unhealthy Fixes
- Psychotherapy
- Prescription Drugs
- Holistic Approaches to Emotional Well-being

At the heart of nearly every transitional woman lies an essential paradox: just at the point when your experience and maturity have given you more confidence and self-esteem than you've ever before possessed, your body starts letting you down. Rather than sailing smoothly along, buoyed by a healthy, energetic, and youthful body, you find you're less physically able to do all you'd like.

Finding Emotional Well-being

Of course, if you've read all the preceding chapters, you know there's lots you can do to maintain your health and vigor. By eating right and exercising, by understanding how to prevent common ailments, and by choosing the right treatment for health problems you can't avoid, you can add years of youthfulness to your life and eventually make a seamless transition into menopause.

Until you put the many suggestions I've offered into practice, you may find the going a little rough. Even after you have taken more control over your physical self, you may not be able to find the total well-being you seek until you come to terms with the emotional and psychological challenges of being a transitional woman.

Still, you can do it! I know because I've seen hundreds of transitional women achieve a much deeper sense of emotional well-being and happiness than they ever felt before. How did they manage? First, by understanding the roadblocks common to the transitional years. Then, by using a variety of effective strategies—all of which I'll discuss in this chapter—to overcome them successfully.

Depression

By the time she was thirty-eight, Janine already had spent many years in the competitive world of fashion design. But after she landed a coveted position as vice president of design for a women's clothing firm, her career took off. She became well respected in the fashion world, and business soared not just because she was talented but also because she was beautiful; everyone said she was the best advertisement for the designs she created.

The world of fashion demands unending youthfulness

from its leaders, a fact Janine took very seriously. Over the years, she frequented spas and underwent several cosmetic surgeries, including a face-lift, a tummy tuck, and liposuction, to keep herself looking young. Actually, she became obsessed with looking youthful.

As she reached her mid-forties, Janine began to feel more and more depressed about what she termed her "fading beauty." She complained of feeling worthless and experiencing enormous fatigue, made worse by frequent insomnia. Her work began to suffer and the upbeat flair she was noted for disappeared from her designs. Before long, sales declined, which led to a less prestigious assignment at her firm and Janine's deepening depression.

Fortunately, Janine's story has a happy ending. She went into counseling, and after many months of hard work, gradually began to accept the inevitability of the physical changes her body was undergoing. She also changed her eating habits and made exercise part of her daily routine, which gave her a physical and emotional lift. Today, she runs her own fashion consulting business, is putting her years of experience and expertise to their best advantage, and feels better than she has in years.

Janine's story shows how depression can sabotage the well-being of an otherwise healthy transitional woman. Over the more than thirty years I've practiced medicine, I've seen depression prevent hundreds of transitional women from enjoying the personal and professional success they've worked so hard to achieve.

Of course, depression doesn't show up in exactly the same way in every individual. This particular malady has a wide range of symptoms, from a lingering case of the blues to a dramatic change in appetite or weight, problems sleeping, fatigue, lethargy, irritability, loss of interest in things you used to enjoy, feelings of worthlessness, self-blame, guilt, difficulty concentrating—even thoughts of death or suicide. No matter how depression affects you, it hurts.

Sometimes depressed people are unaware that their behavior has changed. They also don't realize that they can conquer their feelings of hopelessness. If other people have noticed a change in your outlook, consider whether or not you might be experiencing depression. If it's a possibility, take action to lift yourself out of the doldrums. This is an all-important tack that no one else can do for you.

Anxiety and Panic Attacks

A nervous second cousin to depression, anxiety is also widespread among transitional women and, again, affects each individual in different ways. Symptoms range from occasional feelings of worry and uneasiness to frequent panic attacks, complete with heart palpitations, a tightening of the throat, trembling, sweating, and inescapable feelings of dread. Some people are nervous by nature, but even bold and confident people can be hit by a panic attack with sudden force, as Marina, forty-three, discovered.

A successful image consultant for a beauty products company, Marina managed to make growing older work to her advantage—even in her youth-oriented field—by attracting a client base of thirty-five-plus professional and executive women who saw her as a role model. "If she can look this great at forty-three, then I can, too," is the way one of her clients put it.

Then Marina was asked to work with a group of young saleswomen at one of her firm's out-of-town locations, counseling them on how to take better advantage of their already sensational looks. Several days into these sessions, however, she overheard one twenty-one-year-old complain, "How can I take what Marina says seriously? She's old enough to be my mother. How can she possibly understand what will work for me?"

Instead of laughing off the comment, Marina suffered a full-blown anxiety attack. She started hyperventilating, felt dizzy, and broke into a sweat; her heart began pounding deep in her chest. As soon as the attack passed, she got on the next plane home. Later that week, she confided to me: "All I could think about was that I was too old and washed up to ever work again. I felt so anxious I could have jumped out of that plane!"

Thanks to an understanding boss, Marina didn't lose her job. Her action was blamed on "nervous fatigue" and after a brief vacation she was back at the office. "I'm not myself," she says, however. "Whenever I have to meet with a young client, I get very anxious and panicky. I feel the same each time I look in a mirror; if I find a new gray hair, I freak out." I can attest to that. Every time Marina notices the slightest physical change—from a tiny facial wrinkle to a change in her periods—she comes into my office demanding a series of tests and a great deal of reassurance.

Certainly, Marina is an extreme case; most women don't fly into such an emotional dither. In my experience, however, the vast majority of transitional women do suffer from anxiety for one reason or another. Some are rattled by physical changes caused by growing older. Some are upset by the realization that they are less able to do certain things—conceive a baby, work all day and still party at night—than they were when they were younger. Unless you take steps to discover greater peace of mind, anxiety can become a barrier to happiness during your transitional years.

Premenstrual Syndrome

Even if you take the physical changes in stride, you still may find yourself a bit more testy and moody these days. So what's going on?

It may well be that certain hormonal changes are to blame, particularly if you find yourself at your most depressed and anxious either just before or during your period.

About a week before your period each month, your estrogen and progesterone levels begin to drop—at first gradually, then much more dramatically. In some women, this decline, along with changes in the ratio of estrogen to progesterone, can trigger intense premenstrual mood swings, irritability, depression, and generalized feelings of anxiety known as premenstrual syndrome (PMS). As you reach your early to mid forties, these hormonal shifts grow even more intense—and *that*, in turn, leads to heightened PMS.

(FYI: You'll be glad to hear that PMS usually improves after age forty-five because the dramatic hormonal changes that used to occur with each cycle are less likely. Thus, the emotional shifts ease.)

It's also hypothesized that lower overall estrogen levels may trigger emotional upset during menstruation. When you're in your twenties and early thirties, estrogen stimulates certain catecholamines to become catecholestrogens, compounds that excite particular areas in your brain and reflex system. As estrogen levels decrease in the transitional years, these catecholamines may not get activated. Thus, your brain and reflex system may no longer be stimulated in the same way during your period, resulting in lethargy, sadness, and depression.

The best way to tell if hormones are causing or are at

least aggravating your distress is to chart your symptoms for a couple of months. (Once again, you can use the symptoms diary back on page 32.) If you begin to notice that you're more moody, anxious, and depressed at the same time in your cycle each month, your problem is probably cyclic and, thus, hormone-related. If your symptoms are random, they're most likely caused by a psychosocial problem, which we'll discuss later on in this chapter.

Solving PMS.

The medical community is still stumbling around somewhat in trying to find a "cure" for PMS. But I can tell you what has worked for many of my patients. First, I insist that they follow a healthful diet. Eating more complex carbohydrates such as pasta and whole grains, and cutting down on sugar and caffeine seem to help many transitional women. If the problem is persistent and severe, however, I've found hormone therapy—usually progesterone supplementation—can be very effective.

If your problems get worse *during* your period rather than beforehand, you, too, can try changing your diet. If that doesn't help, speak with your doctor about estrogen and/or estrogen-progesterone supplementation. Very low doses of these hormones can make a world of difference in helping your symptoms to disappear or, at the very least, become more tolerable. (For more detailed information on hormone therapy, see Chapter Three.)

UNDERSTANDING BLOOD SUGAR

Problems with blood sugar levels can also throw you off kilter emotionally. In order for your brain to function effectively, you need to have enough blood sugar in your system. The normal range is about 80 to 105 milligrams per decaliter of glucose in your blood plasma. If your blood sugar drops below this level, your brain doesn't work at its peak, which could cause irritability and lethargy. If your blood sugar level climbs too high above it, you might feel disoriented and moody.

To find out if a blood sugar imbalance is responsible for your upset, your doctor may recommend a few tests, including a simple blood test, possibly followed by a postprandial (after eating) test. Depending upon the outcome, this may be followed by a glucose tolerance test. If your blood sugar levels are only slightly below normal, you may well be able to correct the problem with some simple changes in your diet. Increased intake of complex carbohydrates such as pasta and potatoes, and fruit juice, particularly citrus juices, can help bring blood sugar levels up.

If your sugar level is high—a condition called *diabetes mellitus*—your doctor also will recommend a change in your diet to bring it into the normal range, but this time you will need to *reduce* your intake of carbos and fats. If you don't respond to these dietary changes and you're over forty, you probably have the kind of diabetes (Type 2 diabetes) that commonly responds to oral medications, such as Orinase, DiaBeta, or Diabinese, which is what your doctor will most likely prescribe. These medications promote the release of the hormone insulin from your pancreas, which helps to lower blood sugar levels.

If you have Type 2 diabetes and the medications don't

help, or if you are under forty (in which case you probably have Type 1 diabetes, which does not respond well to oral drugs), your body is simply not able to make enough insulin or to use the insulin it does make to keep blood sugar levels down. In that case, your doctor will prescribe insulin, usually self-administered by injection.

Thyroid Problems

Problems with your thyroid may also affect your emotional well-being. If your thyroid is not active enough, you may feel lethargic and depressed. If it's overactive, you may feel edgy, irritable, and, eventually, very tired. Blood tests can determine whether or not you have a thyroid problem. If you do, chances are good that thyroid medication will offer you relief. (For lots more on the impact of your thyroid, see Chapter Nine.)

Life Demands

We now know that both mind and body play a role in overall well-being. Problems are seldom strictly mental or physical. Psychological troubles can manifest themselves as physical complaints; physical changes can bring emotional upset. What is most important to you as a transitional woman is how you are handling the *whole* picture.

Because the transitional period comprises such a long time—fully fifteen years of your life—chances are you will be struggling to manage a great many pressures during this period. Those stressors vary enormously from woman to woman, reflecting the individuality of transitional women's lives.

Some transitional women, for example, are dealing with the joys, anxieties, and physical demands of pregnancy and first-time motherhood. Others have already gone through that stage, and are busy carpooling school-age kids or trying to cope with the raging hormones and emotional ups and downs of teenage offspring. Still others are becoming grandmothers for the first time! Additionally, many transitional women find that they've become card-carrying members of the "sandwich" generation, at once dealing with the enormous demands of motherhood while coping with their own aging parents, whose increasing frailty may require huge amounts of time, attention, and emotional resilience.

Furthermore, the transitional years seem to be a time when marital infidelities increase. Over and over again, my transitional patients tell me that they've discovered that their husband or live-in partner is having an affair, a situation that wreaks havoc on their emotional well-being. Many also confess their own infidelity, often blaming the indiscretion on their need to have their attractiveness reinforced by a new man who finds them appealing.

As we've discussed in an earlier chapter, problems with sexuality are also common. Some transitional women say that they've lost interest in sex. Others complain about boredom. Those whose mates aren't satisfying them anymore either go on feeling frustrated or turn to outside relationships for satisfaction, which often leads to feelings of guilt, anxiety, and depression.

Single transitional women have their own set of problems. If they're mothers, they're under enormous emotional, physical, and often financial pressure, trying to be mom, dad, and breadwinner all at once. If they have no children, they may feel increasingly desperate to find a parenting partner before their biological clock winds down.

Even if they don't want any (or any more) children, most single transitional women still long for sexual companionship. Once they hit their forties, they may grow more depressed as the available pool of emotionally stable, healthy, heterosexual single males seems to dwindle and opportunities to pair up appear to be few and far between.

Ironically, this perceived lack of available males may be exacerbated by a very healthy sense of self—another common paradox of the transitional years. Because transitional women are more confident in who they are and what they want, they think too highly of themselves to latch onto any guy who comes along. While they may no longer care if he's a ringer for Kevin Costner, they want someone they find sexually attractive. Although they may not demand that he earn lots of money—many transitional women support themselves just fine with their own careers—they want someone who is secure and happy in his work. Today's single transitional woman wants a true helpmate, in every sense of that word. While some women may be anxious and depressed at the thought of "growing old alone," they are nonetheless more and more selective, thus creating a social and emotional bind that can be quite stressful.

By the time you've reached your transitional years, you've had an opportunity to spend at least fifteen years out in the workplace shaping a career. You may even be on your second or even third profession. Many transitional women who have had hard-driving careers come to the realization that there is, indeed, a "glass ceiling" in their company or field and that they may not be able to break through it despite all their years of work.

If hitting the glass ceiling is not enough to trigger emotional distress, try also juggling the demands of families and work, a widespread dilemma of the transitional years. Gail, thirty-nine, a magazine editor, has found this particularly trying. I had recommended to her that she work some exercise into her daily routine when she burst out, "Bernie, it's like this. I dedicated myself to my job for sixteen years. Then, I got married, and because I was already thirty-eight, we decided to have a baby right away. And boy, did things change then. Most days I find myself racing around like a maniac. I get up at five A.M., tend to the baby, wait for the nanny to arrive, race to the train, get to the office, put in eight or nine hours there, rush home, make dinner, then try to spend an hour or two with my daughter before I put her down. Then I read some manuscripts, and fall into bed totally exhausted by ten at night. Sex life? What sex life? Eat right? I'm lucky if I can grab a muffin or slice of pizza in between meetings. Exercise? Get more sleep? You've got to be kidding!"

Sound familiar? Such a fast-paced, pressure-packed life can take a terrible toll on a transitional woman's body. It can also wear you out emotionally. The guilt alone is enough to catapult anyone into a real depression. When you're at work, you feel guilty about not being home. When you're at home, you feel guilty that you're not devoting enough time to the job.

Even if you put your career on hold when the kids are small, the pressures don't diminish; you just feel a different sort of stress, as Cynthia, a thirty-eight-year-old patient, recently explained: "I feel fortunate that I am financially able to take some time out from working to be with my children. But I feel guilty about not bringing in any income, and I feel that some of my working friends look down at me for taking the easy way out. It's also really strange and uncomfortable to have to ask my husband for money when I want to buy something for myself. I mean, I've always had a salary and a career. Now I'm 'just a mom.' I know motherhood is important, but I can't deny that it's also kind of distressing. I also worry about what this will mean for my career in the long run. I do intend to go back to work some day. But will I be obsolete and unwanted by then?"

Unhealthy Fixes

Suppose that you've succumbed to one or many of these stressors, and you're feeling depressed and anxious. So you say to yourself, "Okay, I'm feeling lousy. What would make me feel better?" Well, hardly anyone responds, "What would really make me feel better would be to get to the root of my problem, possibly through psychotherapy." In the real world, you're much more likely to say, "I feel lousy. I'd sure feel better if I ate that half-gallon of chocolate chocolate-chip ice cream in the freezer. What a great idea!" Of course, it isn't, and somewhere deep inside you know that, but you do it anyway because it *does* make you feel better, at least for the moment. It's a quick fix.

Unfortunately, one such fix leads to another—and not only is the original problem still there, but now you've got a new one: the fix itself. Before you know it, you're in the grip of any one of a number of unhealthy ways to deal with the depression and/or anxiety you feel. The most common pathological "fixes" for transitional women are hypochondria, anorexia, gluttony, bulimia, and overexercise.

Hypochondria.

Hypochondria is an obsessive concern with your health, an irrational fear that you're ill despite any and all reassurances from your doctors. While it's hard to know exactly why many transitional women become hypochondriacal, I have a few hypotheses. It may be that they're so worried about growing older that they become hypersensitive to any minor body change or physical problem. It may also be a way to avoid doing the things you don't want to do: you can't have sex with your husband if you're plagued by terrible headaches; you can't exercise if you're always suffering from some body ache or pain. True hypochondriasis can stem from a range of psychological problems that vary widely from person to person.

Allie, a forty-year-old mother of four, is an interesting example of a hypochondriacal transitional woman. Concerned about her four young children, Allie worried obsessively that they were not getting the best education. She would barrage the school board with letters and phone calls demanding that they upgrade the quality of education, but she refused to come to the schools for any meetings. Her reason? Ever since her youngest had entered school, she had suddenly become allergic to the school's air. If she went into the building, she would find it impossible to breathe. Once she required emergency oxygen rescue.

Not one allergist or pulmonary specialist nor a single laboratory test could discover the source of Allie's problem. Even the school's dust was tested, but it proved to be no different from the dust in Allie's own home, which she could tolerate. Allie refused psychiatric help, and the problem persisted throughout her boys' education; she became allergic to whatever school they attended and gradually stopped going out at all. After all the children graduated, Allie started feeling better, and soon after her last son's graduation, she returned to a normal way of life.

Anorexia nervosa.

Anorexia nervosa is an intense fear of becoming obese that endures no matter how thin you are. Even when an anorexic becomes emaciated, she believes she is fat and refuses to try to maintain anything close to an optimal weight. You don't have to look like a skeleton to be anorexic. If your body fat is less than 12 to 14 percent of your weight, you qualify. In extreme cases, victims literally starve themselves to death. Short of that, the condition can bring on several serious medical problems, including:

- *Irregular periods.*
- *Amenorrhea (loss of menstrual periods).*
- *General weakness.*
- *Swelling of feet, ankles, and hands* due to reduced protein in the body.
- *Hypothyroidism (underactive thyroid).*
- *Adrenal gland failure,* which upsets the metabolism and triggers a breakdown of bodily functions resulting in dehydration and breathing and cardiac problems.

Anorexia used to be a problem that cropped up mostly in teenagers and young women who felt pressure to keep up with the crowd and emulate the bone-thin models they saw in teen and fashion magazines. Today, anorexia is appearing more and more frequently in transitional women who try to diet away any hint that they may be growing older and, in their minds, less attractive.

Gluttony.

Extreme overeating, or gluttony, is another quick fix for stress, unhappiness, depression, and anxiety. It backfires, of course, as do most of these "solutions," because it results in enormous weight gain and obesity, which, in turn, makes overeaters even more unhappy and depressed.

Bulimia.

A bulimic compulsively overeats, then forces herself to get rid of that food, usually by vomiting or inducing diarrhea, so as not to gain any weight. Mostly we see this condition in teenage girls and young women, but transitional women, particularly those in their early transitional years, are also vulnerable.

Take my patient Georgette, for instance. The college cheerleader who married the school football hero, she was supposed to live happily ever after. But things didn't turn out quite that way. After she married, she taught school so that her husband could study to become an architect. When he got his degree and joined a successful firm, she became pregnant and quit teaching.

Georgette was thirty-seven when the last of her three children entered school. She had gained an enormous amount of weight over the years, and decided to enroll in a weight-reduction program. She was successful, slimming down to her college weight within the first year. But she still felt fat. She became very worried that the frequent entertaining she did for her husband's clients would not allow her to keep her weight down, and so after each client dinner, she excused herself, went into the bathroom, and forced herself to vomit. Soon, she found herself in a habitual binge-and-purge mode. Eventually, Georgette, encouraged by her concerned husband and kids, sought psychological counseling for her bulimia.

Overexercising.

Kirsten, thirty-six, looked as if she were in great shape. And why not? She ran twice a day—five miles in the morning and ten at night. On the weekends, she spent at least five more hours lifting weights at the local gym. Missing a workout was unthinkable to her; once, she even completed her daily runs with a fever of 103! Exercise was no longer a healthful, enjoyable way for Kirsten to release the stress her job as a corporate lawyer generated—the reason she started exercising in the first place. Exercise—or, more accurately, overexercise—had become an obsession she couldn't kick. Even when such excessive activity caused her to stop menstruating—a condition that was preventing her from conceiving the child she and her husband wanted—she couldn't quit. "I've tried, Bernie," she told me. "But whenever I slow down, I get so edgy and irritable that I just want to jump out of my skin!"

Overexercising is an increasingly common predicament for transitional women. As with all unhealthy fixes, these women (and men) usually begin for the right reasons—to release stress, relax, burn off excess calories. But because exercise works, and is not just socially acceptable but laudable, it can get out of hand. At some point, the cure becomes a new problem.

Clearly, as a transitional woman you are subject to a wide variety of serious stressors, from your changing body to your multiple roles of wife, mother, and working woman. But remember: you're also at a point in your life when you've already weathered some of life's ups and downs, and as a result you have become emotionally stronger and psychologically better prepared to cope with whatever comes your way. So take heart. Once you understand the most effective strategies for dealing with these multifaceted stressors, you can learn to handle them effectively and gracefully during and after your transitional years.

Psychotherapy

The key to finding real peace of mind is not to latch onto a fast fix but to try to change your overall attitude, to learn how to see adversity as a challenge and an opportunity for learning, not as an insurmountable obstacle.

Attitude changes about your self-image, marriage, job, and family responsibilities are critically important. But no matter how bright and intelligent you are, you may just be too close to your problems to be able to solve them without the help of a more objective listener. That's why I recommend talking to a dear and trusted friend, or your minister, priest, or rabbi, even your family doctor or gynecologist, who can help you through your distress.

If the upset you feel is more deep-seated or you've gotten enmeshed in one of the fast fixes I described earlier, you need to turn to a mental health professional—a psychiatrist, psychologist, or psychiatric social worker—who is well trained in helping women, and particularly women of your age and socioeconomic level. Psychotherapy is one of the best ways to feel better because it helps you identify the cause of your stress, then to change or eliminate it by breaking out of destructive habits, adjusting your attitudes, and transforming your stress from a depressing, anxiety-provoking problem to the impetus for positive, healthy action.

Often, you will be successful in identifying the source of your upset and learning how to help yourself after just a few visits to the therapist. Sometimes, however, you may need longer-term treatment. This is a decision that should be made between you and the professional with whom you're working. A major downside: the cost. Private professional psychotherapy is quite expensive, although if you have health insurance your treatment may be partially covered. If you can't afford private therapy, you may be able to find a mental health clinic in your hometown that can provide less expensive but effective treatment.

Prescription Drugs

For some individuals, taking certain prescribed drugs while undergoing psychotherapy is the most effective way to get where they want to go. When taken properly, under the strict supervision of a medical doctor, medications can make you feel stronger and more able to get to the root of your problems more successfully.

Most people lump all drugs intended for depression or anxiety under the category of tranquilizers. Actually, tranquilizers are only one subsection of a group of medications known as psychotropics. These drugs work by triggering or inhibiting certain reactions of the central nervous system, changing the way in which it communicates with the rest of your body so that you feel less depressed or anxious.

Among today's most popularly prescribed antidepressants, or mood elevators, is a new group of drugs that includes Prozac, Paxil, and Zoloft. These medications, technically called "serotonin re-uptake inhibitors," work by blocking the monamine serotonin from acting on the nerves in the brain, the effect of which is to make you feel less down. Although the old standards such as Elavil, Nardil, and Tofranil biochemically work in a different way, all these medications are quite effective in lifting your mood.

However, since the way you react to a particular drug in large part depends upon your own biochemical makeup, medical history, and particular psychological problem, it's sometimes a matter of trial and error before you and your physician hit upon just the right medication and dosage level. Don't give up if the first drug you try doesn't help much; eventually, you and your doctor will find the one that works best for you. Do be aware, however, that any of these medications can cause certain unpleasant side effects, from sleepiness to irregularities in heartbeat. Be sure to notify your doctor immediately if you notice any problems.

For anxiety, your doctor might well prescribe an antianxiety drug such as Xanax, which is particularly effective for panic attacks, or Ativan, Atarax, Valium, or Milltown. But take care: since these drugs are intended to calm you down, they may also make you sleepy and somewhat lethargic, so don't take them when you need to be alert.

One more word of caution: many of these drugs are habit forming. If you take them over a long period of time, you can become addicted; if you suddenly stop taking them, you will experience very unpleasant withdrawal symptoms, such as sweating, muscle cramps, vomiting, and convulsions. I urge you, then, to follow your doctor's directions precisely when it comes to taking—or no longer taking—these drugs.

HOLISTIC APPROACHES TO EMOTIONAL WELL-BEING

Through psychotherapy (with or without medication), you're going to work on changing your attitude and finding the courage to remove some of the causes of your stress. This way you'll improve whatever it is at home, at work, or about yourself that is making you feel less than wonderful. But what can you do to help alleviate the strain you're already experiencing? For many, the answer lies in more holistic approaches that center on relaxing the body and mind.

Meditation.

Over the past several years, meditation has become a well-accepted way to relieve stress and to relax. There's really nothing mysterious about meditation: it simply involves learning to be still with yourself, to live more actively in the moment, to be more alert and energetic as well as more peaceful and serene. Meditation helps you to slow your breathing and thus your heart rate, to relax your muscles, even to change brain wave patterns.

There are many ways to meditate. Depending on what works for you, you can do it sitting up with your back straight, lying down, walking in the woods, jogging down a city street, or washing the dishes after dinner. The best way to approach meditation is to find a beginner's class at your community center or other organization and join in. There are also hundreds of books and audiotapes on meditation, many of which are available at your bookstore or library. Once you begin, however, try to commit to it for at least a few months; it takes some time to feel the effects of regular meditation and to evaluate whether it's right for you.

Visualization and guided imagery.

Closing your eyes and letting yourself visualize a peaceful scene or image for several moments—for instance, lying on a quiet beach and letting a balmy breeze caress your face—

can be a wonderful way to let go of your tensions and relax. Visualization works amazingly well for some individuals; it can slow your heart rate and affect your involuntary nervous system to change the way your body actually works. For instance, it can speed up blood flow to one area of the body while slowing its flow to another.

If you have a hard time doing visualization on your own, you might try guided imagery. Here, someone else—a group leader or a voice on an audiotape—guides you through a particular scene or series of images while you close your eyes, listen, and try to imagine. Most people find guided imagery a lot of fun and a great way to relax.

Hypnosis.

Although a form of guided imagery, hypnosis requires the help of a trained, professional hypnotist. It is a safe and effective way to stay more relaxed and calm.

Progressive muscle relaxation.

When you feel yourself tighten up, a great way to let go is to tense, then relax, one part of your body at a time. This helps you become consciously aware of the tension that has been building in your body. Start with your feet, then move on to the legs, buttocks, abdomen, and so on up your body. It takes only a few minutes and it really does work wonders, particularly if you do it several times a day.

Massage and other bodywork.

Massage is one of the best ways we know to relax the body, releasing muscle tension, improving blood circulation, and making us feel great. A professional masseuse can be a godsend, but a friend or mate skilled in massage techniques can also do the trick.

Other methods of manipulating the body—chiropractic, Rolfing, Feldenkrais, and the Alexander technique—can also help you relax and let go of tension. Just be sure you find a practitioner who is well schooled in his craft; a quack can do your body harm.

Acupuncture and acupressure.

An ancient Chinese therapeutic technique, acupuncture is based on the belief that energy flows throughout the body and that tension, pain, and disease develop where there is a break in the flow. Acupuncturists insert needles at particular points on the body in order to restore a continuous flow of energy, induce healing, encourage relaxation, and promote overall well-being. Acupressure uses similar principles but without the needles.

Yoga.

Yoga involves mastering a series of exercises and postures that require you to focus on your body and your breathing. With yoga you learn to relax areas that are tight to become more flexible. Yoga classes are popping up all over the country, so it's easy and usually inexpensive to enroll. If you don't enjoy classes, try one of the many videotapes on the market. I prefer my patients begin with a class, however, so they can benefit from the personal feedback of a well-trained instructor and learn the basics correctly.

Achieving well-being in your transitional years means many things. You can add years of youthfulness to your life by developing an awareness of your changing body and a new

Finding Emotional Well-being

understanding of how most age-related changes can be prevented, treated, or, at the very least, lived with comfortably. You can face the emotional challenges of the transitional years by learning many techniques that will help you stay calm and serene.

Most of all, you can feel good not only about where you are but where you're headed. Because as a transitional woman, the best part of your life is right within your grasp.

APPENDIX A

Biology 101: The Female Reproductive Cycle

FIGURE A

Your ovaries are two round to oblong-shaped bodies, each about one to one and a half inches long and less than a half inch wide. They lie under the fallopian tubes on each side next to the uterus. When you're born, each ovary contains a half million microscopic cells from which ova, or eggs, will eventually be created. The rest of the ovary is made up of connective tissues that hold it together. Tissues also develop around maturing ova, forming follicles that are responsible for the formation of hormones. The ovaries, then, are the source for both ova and the female hormones estrogen and progesterone.

Appendix A

FIGURE A. *Schematic of Female Reproductive Anatomy*

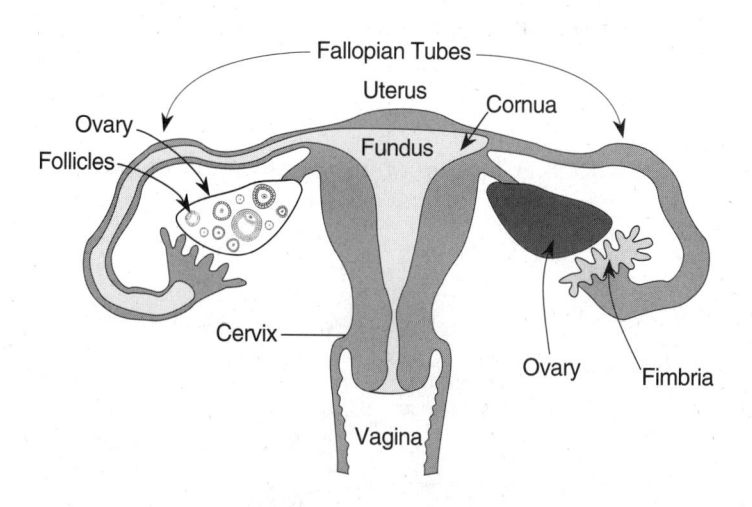

Figure B

About once every eighteen to twenty-six hours from the moment you're born (actually, some scientists think the process begins before birth), an ovum will form spontaneously with cells from the ovary's connective tissue and begin to grow into a follicle. At any given time other eggs are also forming, or have formed, and are of various sizes and in various states of maturity.

As your body first starts to mature sexually (somewhere between the ages of eight and ten), the ovaries begin a series of biochemical events and start to synthesize sex hormones.

While androgens (malelike hormones) are formed first, most of these hormones are converted into the important female hormone estrogen. When enough estrogen becomes available, this triggers changes in your body and sexual organs.

FIGURE B. *Close-up of a Microscopic Section of the Ovary*

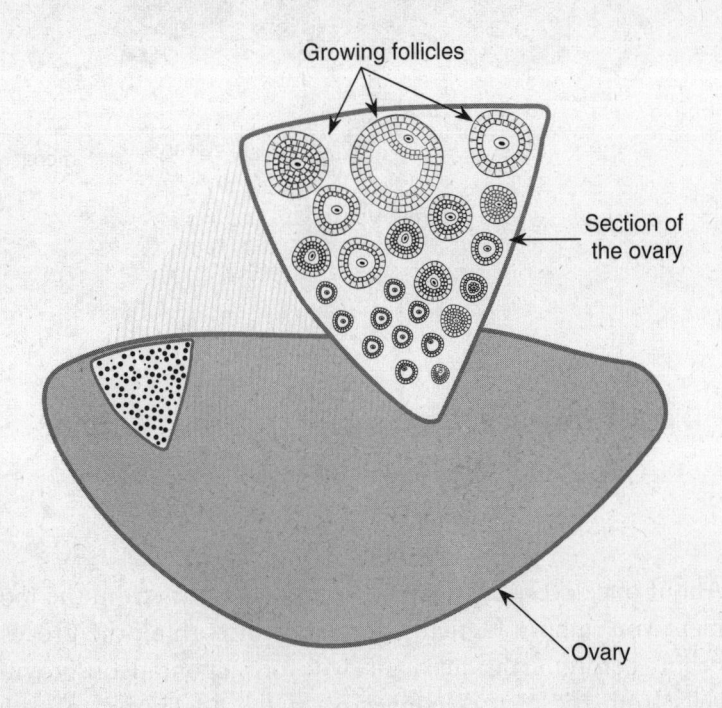

Appendix A

Figure C

At puberty, which occurs somewhere between the ages of eleven and thirteen, brain tissue in the temporal lobe secretes, in a rhythmic manner, a series of chemicals called monamines (MA). Monamines act upon a specific area in the hypothalamus, at the base of the brain, exciting nerve nuclei in a pulsatile manner to produce gonadotropin releasing hormone (GnRH). In turn, GnRH is secreted and eventually reaches the anterior pituitary gland, from which two important pituitary hormones are released: follicle stimulating hormone (FSH) and luteinizing hormone (LH). FSH and LH control the activities within the ovary.

FIGURE C. *Brain-Pituitary-Ovarian Response*

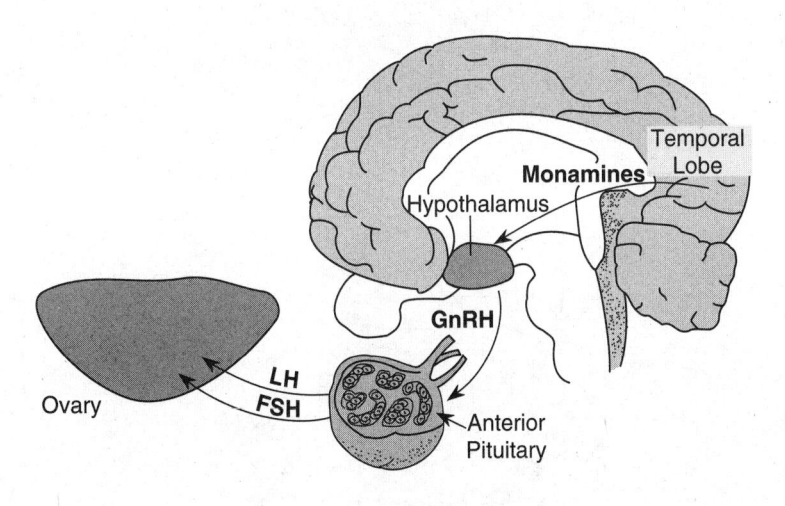

Figure D

FSH and LH regulate the cyclic activity of the ovary, so that usually within eighteen months after your first period a menstrual cycle is established. FSH acts on the follicles to enhance their growth, and causes the most advanced one to become the "dominant follicle." Under FSH's control, this dominant follicle prospers and, with LH levels increasing as well, enlarges. The dominant follicle grows rapidly and by mid-cycle is over an inch in size, so large that it temporarily expands the size of the ovary. Additionally, the cells of all the follicles and tissues produce large amounts of estrogen.

FIGURE D. *Growth of Follicle, and Ovulation*

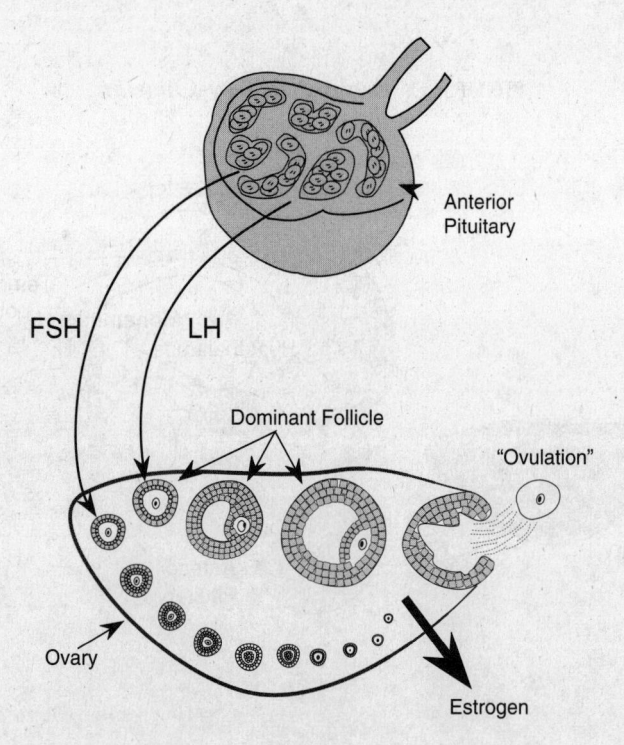

Appendix A

As estrogen levels increase, this signals the pituitary to decrease the amount of FSH released (a process called "negative feedback," because FSH is reduced). This allows better control over the growth of the dominant follicle, which starts to prepare for ovulation. Consequently, LH levels begin to rise. When estrogen reaches its highest level—normally at mid-cycle—it signals the pituitary and hypothalamus to release a large surge of LH (a process called "positive feedback," because LH increases). We believe that this LH surge causes the dominant follicle to rupture and the egg to be thrust out toward the fallopian tube in a shower of fluid. This is called ovulation.

Figure E

The next step takes place in the area of the ovary where the follicle was ruptured. By combining with a fatty substance there, a new body, called the corpus luteum, is formed on

FIGURE E. *Appearance of the Corpus Luteum*

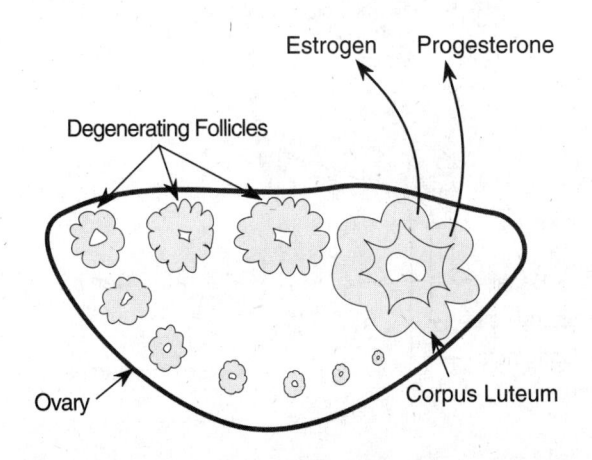

the ovary. The corpus luteum, controlled by LH, has the ability to secrete large amounts of both estrogen and progesterone. The other follicles degenerate (in a process called *atresia*), and the ovaries become relatively dormant for a short time. Now, let's shift our attention to the lining of the uterus.

Figure F

When the ovary began to secrete estrogen, the lining of the uterus (called the endometrium) expanded by first increasing its *basalis* layer. As estrogen increased, a spongy, soft layer,

FIGURE F. *Close-up of the Layers of Endometrium*

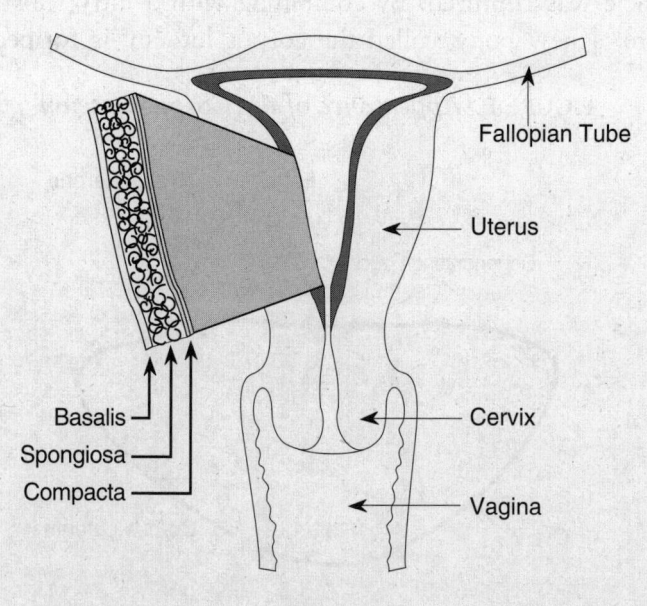

Appendix A

called the *spongiosa*, began to grow on top of the basalis layer. After ovulation, when both estrogen and progesterone became available, a compacting third layer, known as the *compacta*, was added. The compacta protects the other two layers and prepares them to receive the embedded embryo should pregnancy occur. If an egg is fertilized, the embryo comes through the opening of the fallopian tube into the uterus and burrows into these layers of the endometrium, which eventually become the *decidua* (the endometrium in pregnancy).

If pregnancy doesn't occur, the egg is reabsorbed through menstruation, the corpus luteum degenerates in the ovary, hormone levels decrease, and the layers of the endometrium are shed down to the basalis layer again. The sloughing off of these layers results in menstruation. After the initial blood and discarded tissue layers (called *menstruum*) flow out, the uterus clamps down to reduce the blood loss. Toward the end of the period, the revitalization process begins, preparing your body for the next cycle.

APPENDIX B

A Guide to Medical Tests

Test	When and How Often
Absolutely Necessary	
Medical history and physical exam (physician records previous health problems and vital signs, and examines body from head to toe)	Every two years between 35 and 42; yearly from 43 to 50
Breast self-examination	Every month from age 20
Breast exam by doctor	Yearly from 35 to 40; yearly or every six months thereafter
Blood pressure check (detects hypertension)	Yearly
Mammogram (detects early cancer)	Once at 40; every two years until 50; annually thereafter
Pap smear with pelvic exam (detects cancer of the cervix and determines health of reproductive organs)	At least yearly; twice a year recommended particularly if any abnormalities
Rectal exam (detects problems related to reproductive organs as well as hemorrhoids, rectal polyps, or tumors)	Yearly after age 40

Appendix B

Absolutely Necessary (continued)

Stool test (reveals hidden blood in stool specimen and helps detect rectal cancer)	Yearly after age 45

TEST	WHEN AND HOW OFTEN
Highly Recommended	
Electrocardiogram (evaluates current status of heart and may reveal signs of hidden heart disease)	Once between 35 and 40 (baseline); every two years after 40
TSH test (measures thyroid-stimulating hormone in blood to detect thyroid disorders)	Once at 36; every two years thereafter; annually if high risk
Blood sugar check (detects diabetes)	Every two years
Cholesterol check (measures lipid levels in blood to evaluate risk of heart disease)	Every two years until 42; yearly after 42
Complete blood count (detects infection and blood disorders)	Every two years until 42; yearly after 42
Blood chemistry profile (provides information on function of heart, kidneys, liver, and other major body systems)	Every two years until 42; yearly after 42
Complete eye exam (physician measures visual acuity, tests for glaucoma, and evaluates inner eye with ophthalmoscope)	Yearly
Preventive dental checkup (dentist evaluates teeth, gums, and mouth)	Every six months

Sometimes Necessary

Chlamydia culture (detects chlamydia infection, a prevalent STD)	Yearly, if you have more than one sex partner
Dual-photon (X-ray) absorptiometry (measures bone density and may detect early signs of osteoporosis)	Between 35 and 40 if you have a family history or are at high risk for osteoporosis
Podiatric foot exam (provides thorough evaluation of foot problems, including bunions, corns, joint, skin, and circulatory problems)	Between 35 and 40 if you regularly wear high heels or have history of foot pain or problems
FSH test (measures level of follicle-stimulating hormone and confirms menopause is in progress or has occurred)	Discuss this test with your doctor if you're having menopausal symptoms

Promising New Tests for Cancer

Early detection of cancer saves lives. Now, new breakthroughs may make it possible to detect cancer earlier than ever. This is exciting news for all, but especially for those whose family or personal history puts them at greater risk for certain cancers. You'll notice I haven't offered advice on how and when to get these tests; that's because they're not as yet recommended as screening tests for the general public. But they may be soon. Here are a few of the most promising.

CA 125. Detects a cancer antigen (CA 125) that ovarian tumors shed into the blood. This test has been helpful in monitoring the effects of ovarian cancer treatment. In conjunction with other tests, it may also be helpful in monitoring women whose family history puts them at high risk for the disease.

CEA. Measures an antigen in the blood—called carcinoembryonic antigen—that may be elevated in patients with colorectal or certain other cancers. This test also can be useful in monitoring the effectiveness of cancer treatment, but because other diseases can also raise the level of this antigen, it's not yet a useful screening test for cancer.

CA 15-3. A promising blood test used to detect breast cancer recurrence. Clinical trials are being done to assess its value in screening high-risk women.

BIBLIOGRAPHY

CHAPTER ONE
Who Is the Transitional Woman?

Atit, R.; Eskin, B. A.; and Walker, R. F. "Comparison of gonadotropin secretion in women and female rats during aging." *AGE, Journal of the American Aging Association* 9 (1986):10.

Eskin, B. A. "Chapter 1: The menopause and aging." In Eskin, B. A. *Menopause: Comprehensive Management.* 3rd ed. New York: McGraw-Hill, 1994.

Eskin, B. A.; Trivedi, R. A.; Weidemann, C.; and Walker, R. F. "Positive feedback disturbances and infertility in women over 30." *American Journal of Gynecologic Health* 2 (1988):110.

Jacobs, S. L.; Metzger, D. A.; Dodson, W. E.; and Haney, A. F. "Effect of age on response to human menopausal gonadotropin stimulation." *Journal of Clinical Endocrinology and Metabolism* 71 (1990):1525.

Lee, S. J.; Eaton, E. A.; Sexton, L.; and Cooke, I. D. "The effect of age on the cyclical patterns of plasma LH, FSH, oestradiol and progesterone in women with regular menstrual cycles." *Human Reproduction* 3 (1988):851.

Sherman, B., and Korenman, S. G. "Hormonal characteristics of the human menstrual cycle throughout reproductive life." *Journal of Clinical Investigation* 55 (1975):699.

Snowdon, D. A. "Early natural menopause and the duration of postmenopausal life." *Journal of the American Geriatric Society* 38 (1990):402.

Bibliography

CHAPTER TWO
Natural Ways to Maximize Your Vitality

Atkinson, R. L. et al. "Very low-calorie diets (National Task Force on Prevention and Treatment of Obesity)." *Journal of the American Medical Association* 270 (1993):967.
Bulkley, G. B. "Free radicals and other reactive oxygen metabolites: Clinical relevance and the therapeutic efficacy of antioxidant therapy." *Surgery* 113 (1993):479.
Nygaard, E.; Madsen, A. G.; and Christensen, H. "Endurance capacity and longevity in women." *Health Care for Women International* 11 (1990):1–10.
Stanford, J. L. et al. "Factors influencing the age of natural menopause." *Journal of Chronic Disease* 40 (1987):995.

CHAPTER THREE
Coping with Menstrual Changes

Bayer, S. R., and deCherney, A. H. "Clinical manifestations and treatment of dysfunctional uterine bleeding." *Journal of the American Medical Association* 269 (1993):1823.
deZeigler, D., and Bouchard, P. "Understanding endometrial physiology and menstrual disorders in the 1990s." *Current Opinion in Obstetrics and Gynecology* 5 (1993):378.
Eskin, B. A., and Berger, B. "Dysfunctional uterine bleeding in the transitional woman." *The Female Patient* 18 (1993):23.
Fraser, I. S. "Mechanisms of endometrial bleeding." *Reproduction, Fertility and Development* 2 (1990):193.
Hankinson, S. E. et al. "Tubal ligation, hysterectomy and risk of ovarian cancer: a prospective study." *Journal of the American Medical Association* 270 (1993):2813.
Profet, M. "Menstruation as a defense against pathogens transported by sperm." *Quarterly Review of Biology* 68 (1993): 335–81.

Chapter Four
Hot Flashes ... At Your Age?

Brockie, J. A.; Barlow, D. H.; and Rees, M. C. "Menopausal flash symptomatology and sustained reflex vasoconstriction." *Human Reproduction* 6 (1991):472.

Kronenberg, F. "Hot flashes: epidemiology and physiology." *Annals of the New York Academy of Sciences* 592 (1990):52–86.

Rosenberg, J., and Larsen, S. H. "Hypothesis: pathogenesis of postmenopausal hot flush." *Medical Hypotheses* 35 (1991): 349.

Swartzman, L. C.; Edelberg, R.; and Kemmann E. "Impact of stress on objectively recorded menopausal hot flushes and on flush report bias." *Health Psychology* 9 (1990):529.

Chapter Five
Birth Control After Thirty-five

Cramer, D. W., and Cann, C. I. "Risks and benefits of oral contraceptive use in women over 35." *Maturitas*, Supplement 1, (1988):99.

der Simonian, R.; Clemens, J.; Spirtas, R.; and Perlman, J. "Vasectomy and prostate cancer risk: methodological review of the evidence." *Journal of Clinical Epidemiology* 46 (1993):163.

Edgren, R. A. "Oral contraceptives and cancer." *International Journal of Fertility* 36 (1991):37.

Mosher, W. D. "Contraceptive practice in the United States 1982–1988." *Family Planning Perspective* 22 (1990):198–205.

Segal, S. J. et al. "Norplant implants: the mechanism of contraceptive action." *Fertility and Sterility* 56 (1991):273.

Sivin, I. "Dose and age dependent ectopic pregnancy risks with interuterine contraception." *Obstetrics and Gynecology* 78 (1991):291.

Bibliography

Trussell, J. et al. "A guide to interpreting contraceptive efficacy studies." *Obstetrics and Gynecology* 76 (1990):558.

———. "Contraceptive failure in the United States: An update." *Studies on Family Planning* 21 (1990):51.

"WHO collaborative study of neoplasia and steroid contraceptives, breast cancer and combined oral contraceptives (a multinational study)." *British Journal of Cancer* 61 (1990):110.

Wingo, P. A. et al. "Age-specific differences in the relationship between oral contraceptive use and breast cancer." *Obstetrics and Gynecology* 78 (1991):161

Chapter Six
How to Enhance—and Stretch—Your Fertility

Ales, K. L.; Druzin, M. L.; and Santini, D. L. "Impact of advanced maternal age on the outcome of pregnancy." *Surgery, Gynecology and Obstetrics* 171 (1990):209–216.

Edge, V., and Laros, R. K. "Pregnancy outcome in nulliparous women 35 or older." *American Journal of Obstetrics and Gynecology* 168 (1993):1881.

Fonteyn, V. J., and Isada, N. B. "Nongenetic implications of childbearing after age thirty-five." *Obstetrical and Gynecological Survey* 41 (1988):12.

Glassner, M. J.; Aron, E.; and Eskin, B. A. "Clomiphene induction and the rise of heterotopic pregnancies." *Journal of Reproductive Medicine* 35 (1990):175.

Hook, E. B. "Rates of chromosomal abnormalities at different maternal ages." *Obstetrics and Gynecology* 58 (1981):282.

Mansfield, P. K., and McCoal, W. "Toward a better understanding of the advanced maternal age factor." *Health Care for Women International* 10 (1989):395–415.

Milner, M.; Barry-Kinsella, C.; Unwin, A.; and Harrison, R. F. "The impact of maternal age on pregnancy and its outcome."

International Journal of Gynecology and Obstetrics 34 (1992): 281–86.

Naeye, R. L. "Maternal age, obstetric complications, and the outcome of pregnancy." *Obstetrics and Gynecology* 61 (1983): 210.

———. "Maternal body weight and pregnancy outcome." *American Journal of Clinical Nutrition* 52 (1990):273.

Simpson, J. L., and Golbus, M. S. *Genetics in Obstetrics and Gynecology.* 2d ed. Philadelphia: W. B. Saunders Co., 1992.

Spellacy, W. N.; Hondler, A.; and Fene, C. D. "A case control study of 1,253 twin pregnancies from 1982–1987 perinatal data base." *Obstetrics and Gynecology* 75 (1990):168.

Ventura, S. J. "First births to older mothers, 1970–1986." *American Journal of Public Health* 79 (1989):12.

Whittemore, A. S.; Harris, R.; and Itnyre, J. "Characteristics relating to ovarian cancer risk: Collaborative analysis of twelve United States case-control studies." *American Journal of Epidemiology* 136 (1992):1184.

Chapter Seven
How to Enjoy the Best Sex Ever

Cutler, W.; Garcia, C. R.; and McCoy, N. "Perimenopausal sexuality." *Archives of Sexual Behavior* 16 (1987):225.

Dinnerstein, L., and Burrows, G. D. "Hormone replacement therapy and sexuality in women." *Clinics in Endocrinology and Metabolism* 11 (1982):661.

Eskin, B. A. "The transitional woman: sexuality." *Journal of Clinical Practice in Sexuality*, in press.

Leiblum, S., and Bachmann, G. "The sexuality of the climacteric woman." In Eskin, B. A. *Menopause: Comprehensive Management.* Second Edition, New York: Macmillan, 1988.

Shain, R. N.; Miller, W. B.; Holden, A. E.; and Rosenthal, M. "Impact of tubal sterilization and vasectomy on female marital sexuality." *American Journal of Obstetrics and Gynecology* 164 (1991):763–71.

Chapter Eight
Managing Estrogen- and Age-Related Medical Conditions

Anderson, J. J. B., and Metz, J. A. "Contributions of dietary calcium and physical activity to primary prevention of osteoporosis in females." *Journal of the American College of Nutrition* 12 (1993):378.

Barrett-Conner, E., and Kritz-Silverstein, D. "Estrogen replacement therapy and cognitive function in older women." *Journal of the American Medical Association* 269 (1992):2637.

Cowart, B. "Nutrition and chemical aging: Relationships between taste and smell across the adult life span." *Annals of the New York Academy of Science* 561 (1989):39–55.

Cummings, S., and Black, D. "Should perimenopausal women be screened for osteoporosis?" *Annals of Internal Medicine* 104 (1986):817–23.

Ditkoff, E. C.; Crary, W. G.; Cristo, M.; and Lobo, R. A. "Estrogen improves psychological function in asymptomatic postmenopausal women." *Obstetrics and Gynecology* 78 (1991): 991.

Eriksen, E. F., and Kassem, M. "The cellular basis of bone remodeling." *Triangle* 31 (1992):45.

Eskin, B. A. "Malignant potential of benign breast lesions: Implications for estrogen therapy." *Journal of the American Medical Association* 266 (1991):1146.

———. "Chapter 11: The breast in the menopause." In *Menopause: Comprehensive Management*. 3rd ed. New York: McGraw-Hill, 1994.

Gennari, C., and Agnusdei, D. "Calcitonin in bone pain management." *Current Therapy Research* 44 (1988):712–22.

Ghent, W. R., and Eskin, B. A. "Iodine deficiency breast syndrome." In *Frontiers of Thyroidology*. Edited by G. Medeiro-Neto and E. Gaitan. New York: Plenum Press, 1986.

Ghent, W. R.; Eskin, B. A.; Low, D. A.; and Hill, L. P. "Iodine replacement in fibrocystic disease of the breast." *Canadian Journal of Surgery* 36 (1993):453.

Gruber, H. E.; Ivey, J. L.; Baylink, D. J.; et al. "Long-term calcitonin therapy in postmenopausal osteoporosis." *Metabolism* 53 (1984):295–303.

Heinrich, C. H. et al. "Bone mineral content of cyclically menstruating female resistance and endurance trained athletes." *Medicine and Science in Sports and Exercise* 22 (1990):558–63.

Phillips, S. M., and Sherwin, B. B. "Variations in memory function and sex steroid hormones across the menstrual cycle." *Psychoneuroendocrinology* 17 (1992):497.

Spilich, G. J. et al. "Cigarette smoking and cognitive performance." *British Journal of Addiction* 87 (1992):1313.

Wong, M., and Moss, R. L. "Modulation of single unit nerve activity by estrogen priming." *Synapse* 10 (1992):94.

Chapter Nine
The Thyroid: Outsmarting a Midlife Imposter

Eskin, B. A. "The thyroid and sexuality in the menopause." *Journal of Clinical Practice of Sexuality* 7 (1992):6.

Sinks, M. I. et al. "American Thyroid Association guidelines for use of laboratory tests in thyroid disorders." *Journal of the American Medical Association* 263 (1990):1529.

Solomon, B. L.; Glinoer, L. R.; and Wartofsky, L. "Current trends in the management of Graves' disease." *Journal of Clinical Endocrinology and Metabolism* 70 (1990):1518.

Stall, G. M.; Harris, S.; Lokoll, L. J.; and Dawson-Hughes, B. "Accelerated bone loss in hypothyroid patients overtreated with 1-thyroxine." *Annals of Internal Medicine* 113 (1990): 265.

Volpe, R. "Immunology of human autoimmune thyroid disease."

Bibliography

In *Autoimmune Disease of the Endocrine System*. Boca Raton, Fla.: CRC Press, 1990.

CHAPTER TEN
Beating Serious Illness

Appel, L., and Bush, T. "Preventing heart disease in women." *Journal of the American Medical Association* 266 (1991):565.

Barrett-Conner, E. "Diabetes, hypertriglycerdemia and heart disease risk in women." *International Journal of Fertility* 37, Supplement 2 (1992):72–82.

Eskin, B. A.; Snyder, D. L.; and Roberts, J. "Protective action of female sex hormones on adrenergic neurotransmission in the aging female heart." *Proceedings of the American Fertility Society* 48 (1992):89.

Gurwitz, J. H.; Nananda, F.; and Avorn, J. "The exclusion of the elderly and women from clinical trials in acute myocardial infarction." *Journal of the American Medical Association* 268 (1992):1417.

King, M-C.; Rowell, S.; and Love, S. M. "Inherited breast and ovarian cancer." *Journal of the American Medical Association* 269 (1993):1975.

Kritz-Silverstein, D.; Wingard, D. L.; and Barrett-Connor, E. "Employment status and heart disease risk factors in middle-aged women: The Rancho Bernardo Study." *American Journal of Public Health* 82 (1992):215–19.

Miller, B. A. et al. "Recent incidence trends for breast cancer in women and the relevance of early detection: An update." *CANCER* 43 (1993):27.

Skobeloff, E. M. et al. "The influence of age and sex on asthma admissions." *Journal of the American Medical Association* 268 (1992):3437.

Wingard, D. L. et al. "Sex differentials in morbidity and mortality risks examined by age and cause in the same cohort." *American Journal of Epidemiology* 130 (1989):601–610.

Wu, M. L. et al. "Personal and environmental characteristics related to epithelial ovarian cancer, I. Reproductive and menstrual events and oral contraceptive use." *American Journal of Epidemiology* 128 (1988):1216.

CHAPTER ELEVEN
A Doctor's Guide to Looking Good

Bazzano, G. et al. "Effect of retinoids on follicular cells." *Journal of Investigative Dermatology* 101 (1993):138S.

Weiss, M. A.; Weiss, R. A.; and Goldman, M. P. "How minor varicosities cause leg pain." *Contemporary Obstetrics/Gynecology* 36 (1991):113–25.

Yaer, M., and Gilcrest, B. A. "Cellular and molecular mechanisms of cutaneous aging." *Journal of Dermatologic Surgery and Oncology* 16 (1990):915.

CHAPTER TWELVE
Finding Emotional Well-being

Crofford, O. B., and the Diabetes Control and Complications Trial Research Group. "The effect of intensive treatment of diabetes." *New England Journal of Medicine* 329 (1993):977.

Eskin, B. A. "The thyroid and sexuality in the menopause." *Journal of Clinical Sexuality* 7 (1992):6.

Phillips, S. M., and Sherwin, B. B. "Effect of estrogen on memory function in surgically menopausal women." *Psychoneuroendocrinology* 17 (1992):485.

Rigotti, N. A. et al. "The clinical course of osteoporosis in anorexic women." *Journal of the American Medical Association* 265 (1991):1133.

Surgeon General Report. "The health benefits of smoking cessation." Department of Health and Human Services. Publication #CDC 90-8416 (1990):371–423.

Index

acquired immune deficiency syndrome (AIDS), 36, 108, 167, 171, 179–80
acupuncture and acupressure, 304
adult acne, 271–73
age and aging, 291
 changes you may experience with, 17–21
 and estrogen, 13–16
 and FCD, 192–98
 intensity of transitional symptoms with, 16–17
 medical conditions related to, 191–214
 and NAS, 20–21, 192, 206–14
 and osteoporosis, 192, 198–205
 and physical appearance, 264, 266, 280–81
 and thyroid disorders, 21, 216
alcohol, 42–43, 202, 251
allergic edema, 245–47
alphahydroxy acids (AHAs), 269
amenorrhea, 53, 296
American Fertility Society, 151–54
American Heart Association, 235, 237, 242
androgens, 160–61, 274, 308
androstenedione, 259
anemia, 50, 54, 71
anorexia nervosa, 296
anti-anxiety drugs, 301
antidepressants, 98, 176, 300–301
 hot flashes and, 77, 86–87
 for memory enhancement, 212
anti-estrogen drugs, 164, 197, 255
 hot flashes and, 85–86
antihistamines, 210–11, 249
anti-hot flash drugs, 96–98
antioxidants, 41–42, 56
anti-prostaglandins, 197
anxiety and panic attacks, 285–88, 291–92, 294, 296, 299–301
artery and vein problems, 244–47
 allergic edema, 245–47
 spider veins, 277
 thrombophlebitis, 60, 244–45, 278
 varicose veins, 278–79
artificial insemination, 123, 148, 150–51
Artificial Insemination Homologous (AIH), 150–51
assisted reproductive technologies (ART), 141, 152
athletic supporters, 147

barrier contraceptives, 106–8
basal body temperature:
 birth control and, 113–14
 fertility and, 132–36, 139, 141–42
Bellergal-S, 97–98
Bernie's Ten-Point Plan for Health and Vitality, 30–47
 and avoiding unnecessary gynecological surgery, 43–45

Index

Bernie's Ten-Point Plan for Health and Vitality (*continued*)
  and common symptoms of transitional years, 30–31
  and keeping track of premenopausal symptoms, 31–33
  and maintaining optimal weight, 37–42
  and noninvasive wellness tests, 46–47
  and sex, 31–37
  and smoking, alcohol, and caffeine, 42–43
  and STDs, 34–36
  and stress, 39, 45
  and thyroid checkups, 33–34
biphosphonates, 204
birth control:
  and avoiding surprise pregnancies, 118–19
  barrier methods of, 106–8
  and downside of pregnancy and childbearing in later life, 101–6
  implants and, 110–11
  injections and, 109–10
  IUDs and, 111–13
  for men, 108–9, 117–18, 167–68
  natural methods of, 113–14
  surgical approaches to, 114–18
  after thirty-five, 100–119
birth control pills (BCP), 109
  cancer and, 60–62, 92, 251, 257, 259
  downside of, 59–60
  endometriosis and, 175
  guidelines for taking, 63
  for hot flashes, 91–94
  menstruation and, 50, 58–63, 65, 70, 72, 92–93, 109
  ovarian cysts and, 129
  progesterone therapy and, 65
  sexual enjoyment and, 176
  who should not take them, 62

bleaching, 276
blood sugar, 289–90
bones, 12, 49
  and Bernie's Ten-Point Plan for Health and Vitality, 37, 39–40
  loss of, 20, 39
  NAS and, 209
  and pregnancy in later life, 101
  see also osteoporosis
boredom, sexual enjoyment and, 180
breast cancer, 111, 235, 250–55
  anti-estrogens and, 85
  and anti-hot flash drugs, 97
  BCP and, 61–62
  detection of, 46, 252–54
  FCD and, 194–95
  and pregnancy in twenties, 101
  progesterone therapy and, 96
  reducing risk of, 251–52
  treatment of, 254–55
breasts:
  and Bernie's Ten-Point Plan for Health and Vitality, 31–33
  estrogen and, 14
  FCD and, 192–98, 250
  Norplant and, 110
  PMS and, 6, 21, 72–73
  progesterone therapy and, 65, 95
  sagging of, 10, 43, 264
  self-examinations of, 63
Brigham and Women's Hospital, 116, 235
bromergocryptine, 144
bulimia, 297

caffeine, 42–43, 196
calcium, 20
  osteoporosis and, 199–203, 205
cancer, 7, 94, 249–62
  BCP and, 60–62, 92
  and Bernie's Ten-Point Plan for Health and Vitality, 41–42, 44–45
  menstrual changes and, 50, 53–54, 60–62, 64, 67–68, 75

Index

promising new tests for, 316–17
thyroid disorders and, 226–27, 232
treating it after thirty-five, 261–62
see also specific kinds of cancer
Candida, 165–66
catecholamines, 206–7, 287
cell activity, aging and, 13–14
cerebral vascular accidents (CVAs), 238
cervical cancer, 255–56
   IUDs and, 113
   prepregnancy checkups and, 131
   sexual enjoyment and, 173
cervical caps, 107–8
cervical mucus, 114
   fertility and, 136, 148, 150, 152
chemotherapy, 28, 173, 261
   gynecological cancers and, 254, 256–57
chlamydia, 34–35, 125, 168–69
cholesterol, 14
   heart disease and, 236, 241
   progesterone therapy and, 65–66
   thyroid disorders and, 218
chronic illness, sexual enjoyment and, 174–75
clomiphene and clomiphene citrate, 85, 122–23, 140, 143, 150
clonidine, 87, 96–97
collagen injections, 270
condoms, 108–9, 167–68
contraceptive foam and inserts, 107
contraceptive sponges, 107
cosmetic surgery, 270–71, 284

Dalkon Shield, 111
danazol, 85–86
depilatories, 276
Depo-Provera, 109–10
depression, 9, 16, 33
   emotional well-being and, 283–85, 287–88, 291–94, 296–97, 299–300
   PMS and, 21

and pregnancy later in life, 103
and psychological and psychosocial changes, 23
thyroid disorders and, 217, 231
dermabrasion, 270
diabetes, 244
   emotional well-being and, 289–90
   gynecological cancers and, 257
   heart disease and, 239–40
diaphragms, 106–7
diet, 4–5
   and Bernie's Ten-Point Plan for Health and Vitality, 30–31, 37, 40–41
   emotional well-being and, 283–84, 288–89
   fruits and vegetables in, 40–41
   grains and cereals in, 41
   gynecological cancers and, 251–52, 259–60
   heart and, 241
   hot flashes and, 19, 89
   menstrual changes and, 50, 56–57, 66, 72
   milk and dairy products in, 41
   NAS and, 209, 214
   osteoporosis and, 202–3, 205
   physical appearance and, 266, 273, 279
   protein foods in, 41
   and risk of early menopause, 26, 29
dilation and curettage (D&C), 44–45, 54, 75, 164, 222
donor egg IVF, 154

echocardiograms, 240–41
ectopic pregnancy, 127, 155
electrolysis, 277
emollients, 267
emotional well-being, 282–305
   and anxiety and panic attacks, 285–88, 291–92, 294, 296, 299–301
   blood sugar and, 289–90

Index

emotional well-being *(continued)*
  depression and, 283–85, 287–88, 291–94, 296–97, 299–300
  holistic approaches to, 301–4
  life demands and, 290–94
  medication and, 289–90, 300–301
  PMS and, 287–88
  psychotherapy for, 299–302
  sex and, 177–81, 291–93
  thyroid problems and, 290
  unhealthy fixes and, 294–99
endometrial biopsies, 164
endometrial cancer, 64
endometrial sampling, 142
endometriosis:
  fertility and, 139–41
  sexual enjoyment and, 175–76
erection loss, 187
ergotamine drugs, 97
estrogen, 20
  aging and, 13–16
  and anti-hot flash drugs, 97–98
  and artery and vein problems, 246–47
  BCP and, 58–61
  and Bernie's Ten-Point Plan for Health and Vitality, 34–36, 40, 42–43
  and decreasing effectiveness of ovaries, 11, 14–16
  emotional well-being and, 287–88
  FCD and, 192–98
  in female reproductive cycle, 306, 308, 310–13
  fertility and, 142, 154
  gynecological cancers and, 250–51, 258–59
  heart disease and, 236–38
  hot flashes and, 16, 66, 78–79, 83–88, 92–96, 98
  lifetime levels of, 14–15
  management of, 191–99, 201, 204–11
  menstrual changes and, 50–53, 57–63, 66–70, 72–75
  NAS and, 192, 206–11
  osteoporosis and, 192, 199, 201, 204–5
  physical appearance and, 272, 274, 276
  PMS and, 16, 21, 66
  pulmonary problems and, 248
  sexual enjoyment and, 160–64
  thyroid disorders and, 21, 222, 224, 227
  tubal ligations and, 115
estrogen replacement therapy (ERT), 262
  cancer and, 61, 258–59
  menstrual changes and, 57, 61, 67, 74
  sexual enjoyment and, 174
estrogen supplement therapy (EST):
  guidelines for successful, 68–69
  hot flashes and, 78–79, 93–95
  menstrual changes and, 66–69
  NAS and, 208, 211
  who should not use it, 67
exercise, 5, 239
  aging and, 13
  and Bernie's Ten-Point Plan for Health and Vitality, 30–31, 38–39
  emotional well-being and, 283–84, 293, 298–99, 304
  fertility and, 129
  heart and, 242–43
  hot flashes and, 19, 91
  Kegel, 163
  menstrual changes and, 50, 55, 66
  NAS and, 209–10
  osteoporosis and, 200, 203
  overdoing it, 298–99
  and risk of early menopause, 27
  varicose veins and, 278–79
exfoliants, 266
eyes, 263–64
  thyroid disorders and, 215, 217–18

Index

face:
  dryness of, 21
  hair on, 22, 25, 74, 95
falloposcopy, 139
fantasy loss, 187–88
female reproductive cycle, 306–13
fertility, 7–8, 126
  aging and, 21
  and amount of time you have left, 121–23
  and Bernie's Ten-Point Plan for Health and Vitality, 33, 36–37, 39–40, 42
  and checking and correcting your anatomy, 136–41
  and conceiving natural way, 132–36
  and difficulty getting pregnant in later life, 124–26
  enhancing and stretching of, 120–57
  and high-tech solutions to problems with, 150–55
  and inability to give birth, 156–57
  male infertility and, 126, 145–50
  menstruation and, 51, 71–72, 133, 140–45
  ovaries and, 11, 124–29, 136, 141–43, 153
  prepregnancy checkups and, 131–32
  protection of, 126–30
  sex and, 130, 133–35, 137–38, 147, 151, 177
  STDs and, 125–26, 168
  thyroid and, 220, 222, 227
fertility drugs, 143–45
fibrocystic breast disease (FCD), 192–98, 250
fibroids (myomas), 86
  fertility and, 138–39, 141
  menstrual changes and, 50, 54
  sexual enjoyment and, 164–65
  unnecessary surgery on, 43–45

follicle-stimulating hormone (FSH), 16, 86
  in female reproductive cycle, 309–11
  fertility and, 142–43, 148–50
  menstrual changes and, 73
  thyroid disorders and, 223–24

gamete intrafallopian transfer (GIFT), 154
Gardnerella vaginalis, 34, 166
glucose tolerance tests, 289
gluttony, 296–97
goiters, 225, 233
gonadotropin-releasing hormone (GnRH), 143–44, 309
gonadotropin-releasing hormone (GnRH) agonists, 86, 176
gonorrhea, 34–35, 125, 168
gums, protection of, 280–81
gynecological surgeries, 4
  damage from, 125–26
  sexual enjoyment and, 172–74
  unnecessary, 43–45
  see also specific gynecological surgeries

hair, 14, 274–77, 286
  coloring of, 275–76
  dryness of, 12
  on face, 22, 25, 74, 95
  graying of, 5, 9
  improving appearance of, 274–77
  thyroid disorders and, 215, 217, 233
headaches, 206–8, 210–11, 213–14
heart:
  and Bernie's Ten-Point Plan for Health and Vitality, 39, 41–42
  keeping it healthy, 240–43
heart disease, 4, 235–43
  BCP and, 60, 62
  risk factors for, 236–40
  treatment of, 243
herpes simplex virus (HSV), 167

Index

high density lipoproteins (HDLs), 236–38, 241
hot flashes, 13, 22, 25, 76–99
  aging and, 17–19
  and Bernie's Ten-Point Plan for Health and Vitality, 35, 37, 44–45
  causes of, 83–89
  estrogen and, 16, 66, 78–79, 83–88, 92–96, 98
  hormone replacement therapy for, 91–98
  impersonators of, 88–89
  medications and, 19, 77, 84–87
  menstruation and, 66, 73, 76–79, 84, 86, 92–96
  number of, 82–83
  osteoporosis and, 205
  ovaries and, 11, 78, 87–88
  simple treatments for, 89–91
  and staying cool, 90
  stress and, 77–78, 81, 87, 90
  symptoms accompanying, 80–81
  tubal ligations and, 114–15
  weight loss and, 84
  what they are, 80–82
  who gets them, 79–80
hot tubs, 146
Huhner's tests, 137
human chorionic gonadotropin (HCG), 123, 143
human immunodeficiency virus (HIV), 151, 167, 170
human papilloma virus (HPV), 167–68
hypertension (high blood pressure), 238–39, 257
hyperthyroidism, 216, 220–27, 296
  osteoporosis and, 202
  symptom checklist for, 218
  treatment of, 229–31
hypnosis, 303
hypochondria, 294–95
hypothalamus, 16, 83, 87, 90

hypothyroidism, 21, 33–34, 216–23, 226–29, 231–33
  symptom checklist for, 217–18
  treatment of, 227–29
hysterectomies, 165, 222
  gynecological cancers and, 256–58
  sexual enjoyment and, 172–73
  unnecessary, 43–45
hysterosalpingograms (HSGs), 137–38, 140
hysteroscopy, 44, 138–39

infections, sex and, 165–71
infertility, *see* fertility
infidelity, 170, 178–79, 291
intracervical insemination (ICI), 151–52
intrauterine devices (IUDs), 111–13
intrauterine insemination (IUI), 151–52
in vitro fertilization (IVF), 153–55
iodine therapy, 197–98
iron, 237–38

Karmali, Rashida, 251–52
Kegel exercises, 163
Kronenberg, Fredi, 79

laparoscopy, 115–16, 260
  diagnostic, 138–40
  fertility and, 153–54
  sexual enjoyment and, 175–76
laparotomies, 115–16, 141
levonorgestrel implants, 110
lithium, 233
liver, 42–43, 94, 96, 111
  EST and, 67–68
  osteoporosis and, 199, 204
low density lipoproteins (LDLs), 236–38, 241
lumpectomies, 254
lung cancer, 248
Lupron, 86
luteinizing hormone (LH), 86

332

Index

in female reproductive cycle, 309–12
  fertility and, 133, 142–43, 148–50
  menstrual changes and, 52, 73

malignant melanomas, 261
mammograms, 46, 63, 252–53
  FCD and, 193–95
marriage, 23
  emotional well-being and, 291–93, 297–99
  infidelity in, 170, 178–79, 291
  sexual enjoyment and, 159
massage, 303–4
mastectomies, 173, 252, 254
masturbation, 163, 189
Medical College of Pennsylvania, 7, 66, 220, 237
medical tests, guide to, 314–17
medication:
  adult acne and, 272–73
  for artery and vein problems, 245, 247
  and Bernie's Ten-Point Plan for Health and Vitality, 44
  and coping with menstrual changes, 55, 64–65, 71
  emotional well-being and, 289–90, 300–301
  for FCD, 197
  heart and, 241, 243
  hot flashes and, 19, 77, 84–87
  male infertility and, 148
  for NAS, 210–11
  for osteoporosis, 204
  for pulmonary problems, 249
  sexuality and, 171–72, 176, 188–89
  for thyroid disorders, 224, 227–30
  see also specific medications
meditation, 302
medroxyprogesterone acetate (MPA), 64–65
memory loss, 16
  aging and, 20–21

NAS and, 207–8, 211–14
thyroid disorders and, 217
men:
  birth control for, 108–9, 117–18, 167–68
  heart disease in, 235–37, 240
  infertility in, 126, 145–50
  sexual problems of, 186–89
menopause, 3–4, 7, 10–13, 19, 22
  BCP and, 92, 109
  and Bernie's Ten-Point Plan for Health and Vitality, 30–33, 43–45
  determining risk of early onset of, 26–30
  endometriosis and, 176
  estrogen and, 14, 16, 68–69
  FCD and, 194
  fertility and, 124, 153–54
  gynecological cancers and, 250, 258–59
  heart disease and, 236, 239–40
  hot flashes and, 76–80, 82–84, 92–93, 95, 97
  menstrual changes and, 49, 73–74
  NAS and, 208
  osteoporosis and, 199
  physiological preparations for, 11, 25
  thyroid disorders and, 216, 222–23, 231
  tubal ligations and, 115–16
menorrhagia, 48–49
menstruation, 261, 313
  adult acne and, 271
  alleviating troublesome symptoms in, 54–57
  and artery and vein problems, 246–47
  BCP and, 50, 58–63, 65, 70, 72, 92–93, 109
  and Bernie's Ten-Point Plan for Health and Vitality, 33, 37, 40, 43, 45
  birth control and, 119

Index

menstruation (*continued*)
  changes in, 6–8, 9, 12–13, 16, 19, 22, 25, 37, 40, 43, 45, 48–75
  diet and, 50, 56–57, 66, 72
  early bleeding or spotting in, 52
  emotional well-being and, 286–88, 296
  endometriosis and, 175
  EST and, 66–69
  exercise and, 50, 55, 66
  FCD and, 192–94
  fertility and, 51, 71–72, 133, 140–45
  good sex and, 57
  gynecological cancers and, 250, 256–57, 260
  heart disease and, 238, 242–43
  home remedies and, 56
  hot flashes and, 66, 73, 76–79, 84, 86, 92–96
  mid-cycle spotting and, 53–54, 74–75
  osteoporosis and, 202
  ovarian cysts and, 128
  persistent spotting and, 53
  progesterone and, 51, 58, 62–66, 70–71, 73–75
  and real-life problems and remedies, 69–75
  and risk of early menopause, 26
  and shorter periods with less flow or no period at all, 52–53, 72–74
  thyroid disorders and, 217–18, 222, 224
  tubal ligations and, 115
  unusually heavy bleeding in, 50–51, 71
  variable bleeding in, 51–52, 69–70
  see also premenstrual syndrome
metabolism, 38–39, 88, 219
methimazole (Tapazole), 229
metronidazole, 167
midlife, definitions of, 10
mini-laparotomies, 115–16

miscarriages, 102, 127, 130
  fertility and, 153, 155
  sexual enjoyment and, 178
  thyroid disorders and, 223
mitral valve prolapse, 174–75
monamines (MA), 309
multiple births, 144–45, 155
muscles, 39
  aging and, 13–14, 19–20
  decline in tone and strength of, 12–13
  emotional well-being and, 302–3
  hot flashes and, 90
  NAS and, 209–10
  and pregnancy in later life, 101–2
mycoplasmosis, 168–69
mycostatins, 166
myomectomies, 44, 164–65

National Cancer Institute, 145, 253, 255
Neurogenic Aging Symptoms (NAS), 20–21, 192, 206–14
  memory loss and, 207–8, 211–14
  remedies for, 210–12
  symptoms of, 206–10
  taking action on, 213–14
nicotine replacement therapy, 243
night sweats, *see* hot flashes
nongenital sensate focus, 185, 189
Norplant, 110–11
nutrition, *see* diet

obesity, 239
oligomenorrhea, 53
omega-3 acids, 251–52
oophorectomies, 258–59
orgasms, 180–81, 183–84
osteoporosis, 4, 40, 192, 198–205
  causes of, 200–202
  Depo-Provera and, 110
  prevention of, 203
  risk of, 199–200
  treatment of, 204–5
ovarian cancer:

Index

anti-hot flash drugs and, 97
BCP and, 61
detection of, 260
fertility drugs and, 145
reducing risk of, 258–60
tubal ligations and, 116
ovarian cysts, 128–29
ovaries, 40
   BCP and, 92
   decrease in effectiveness of, 11, 14–16
   in female reproductive cycle, 306–10, 312
   fertility and, 11, 124–29, 136, 141–43, 153
   hot flashes and, 11, 78, 87–88
   keeping them healthy and intact, 127–29
   menstrual changes and, 49–51, 69, 73
   radiation treatment and, 261–62
   and risk of early menopause, 28
   sexual enjoyment and, 160, 173, 176
   thyroid and, 220, 223
   tubal ligations and, 116
overexercising, 298–99
ovulation:
   birth control and, 110, 113–14
   estrogen and, 15, 95
   FCD and, 192–93
   in female reproductive cycle, 311, 313
   fertility and, 122–25, 127, 130, 133, 140–44
   hot flashes and, 95
   irregular, 125
   menstrual changes and, 51–54, 63–65, 69, 72–73, 75
   progesterone therapy and, 63–65
   thyroid and, 220

Pap smears, 31, 62, 74, 113, 131, 255
pelvic exams, 31

pelvic inflammatory disease (PID):
   and artery and vein problems, 244–45
   fertility and, 125, 127–28
   IUDs and, 112–13
   sexual enjoyment and, 170–71
physical appearance, 263–81
   of hair, 274–77
   and protecting your smile, 280–81
   spider veins and, 277
   varicose veins and, 278–79
   younger-looking skin and, 264–71
pituitary gland, 39, 49
   estrogen and, 16, 67
   in female reproductive cycle, 309, 311
   fertility and, 133, 143–44
   hot flashes and, 88
   menstrual changes and, 52, 67
   thyroid and, 219–20, 223
polyps, 139
positron emission tomography (PET) tests, 240–41
postcoital tests, 137
postpartum blues, 220–21
postpartum thyroiditis, 221, 224, 227
preeclampsia, 102, 144
pregnancy, 9, 23, 313
   avoiding surprise, 118–19
   BCP and, 62, 92
   and Bernie's Ten-Point Plan for Health and Vitality, 40, 42
   checkups prior to, 131–32
   difficulty in, 21, 23, 124–26
   estrogen and, 94–95
   and finding emotional well-being, 291, 293, 297–98
   gynecological cancers and, 250
   in later life, 101–6
   menstrual changes and, 51, 58, 64–65, 71, 73
   osteoporosis and, 200
   progesterone therapy and, 64–65, 96

Index

pregnancy (*continued*)
  radiation treatment and, 261
  and risk of early menopause, 27
  sexual enjoyment and, 177–78, 181
  thyroid disorders and, 217, 220, 223
  see also birth control; fertility
premature ejaculation, 187, 189
premenstrual syndrome (PMS), 6
  aging and, 17–19, 21
  BCP and, 109
  emotional well-being and, 287–88
  estrogen and, 16, 21, 66
  menstrual changes and, 66, 72–73
presbyopia, 13–14
progesterone and progesterone therapy, 62–67
  and adult acne, 272
  and bone loss, 20
  drawbacks of, 65–66
  and emotional well-being, 287–88
  and FCD, 192–93, 197
  in female reproductive cycle, 306, 312–13
  and fertility, 122, 142, 154
  and hot flashes, 92, 94–96
  and IUDs, 111
  and menstrual changes, 51, 58, 62–66, 70–71, 73–75
  and Norplant, 110
  and osteoporosis, 201–2, 205
  possible side effects of, 95
  and sexual enjoyment, 176
  and tubal ligations, 115
progressive muscle relaxation, 303
propylthiouracil (PTU), 229
psychological and psychosocial changes, 22–24
psychological counseling:
  emotional well-being and, 299–302
  sexual enjoyment and, 186, 189
pulmonary problems, 247–49

radiation, 28, 261–62
  gynecological cancers and, 252, 254, 256–57
  sexual enjoyment and, 173
  thyroid disorders and, 232
radioactive iodine therapy, 230
radioactive iodine uptake tests, 226–27
relaxation, 90, 182, 302–4
reproductive organs, damage to, 125–26
Retin-A (tretinoin), 269–70, 273
Roberts, Jay, 237

sclerotherapy, 277
semen, fertility and, 148
senses, heightening or dulling of, 208
serotonin, 86–87
sex and sexuality, 7–8, 12, 23, 57
  and Bernie's Ten-Point Plan for Health and Vitality, 31–37
  and chronic illnesses, 174–75
  diminishing drive for, 7, 10, 21
  and emotional well-being, 177–81, 291–93
  and endometriosis, 175–76
  enjoyment of, 35–37, 57, 158–90
  and experimentation, 184
  and expressing your needs, 183
  and female reproductive cycle, 307–8
  and fertility, 130, 133–35, 137–38, 147, 151, 177
  and gynecological abnormalities, 163–72
  and gynecological surgeries, 172–74
  lubricants used during, 147
  making time for, 182–83
  and medication, 171–72, 176, 188–89
  and men's problems, 186–89
  and physical problems interfering with intimacy, 159–63

Index

and psychological counseling, 186, 189
and risk of early menopause, 29
and sex therapists, 185, 189
and simplifying your life, 182
spicing it up, 181–86
stages of pleasure in, 160
and taking vacations, 181–82
and thyroid disorders, 217, 220–24
and worrying about orgasms, 180–81, 183–84
see also birth control
sexual dysphoria, 187
sexually transmitted diseases (STDs):
  bacterial, 168–69
  and Bernie's Ten-Point Plan for Health and Vitality, 34–36
  birth control and, 107–9
  fertility and, 125–26, 168
  gynecological cancers and, 256
  and risk of early menopause, 29
  sexual enjoyment and, 167–71
  symptoms of, 169
  viral, 167–68
  see also specific sexually transmitted diseases
shampoos, 275
shaving, 277
skin, 7, 14, 263–73
  adult acne and, 271–73
  atrophism of, 265
  dryness of, 12, 16, 21, 43, 215, 217, 263, 266
  pressure on, 268
  thyroid disorders and, 215, 217, 233
  younger-looking, 264–71
smoking, 26, 62, 94, 127, 245
  and Bernie's Ten-Point Plan for Health and Vitality, 42–43
  gynecological cancers and, 251, 256
  heart disease and, 239, 242–43
  osteoporosis and, 202

physical appearance and, 268
Snyder, Dave, 237
spider veins, 277
stamina, 23
  aging and, 19–20
  and Bernie's Ten-Point Plan for Health and Vitality, 34, 40
  emotional well-being and, 284–85, 287
  NAS and, 209, 212–14
  thyroid disorders and, 215, 217–18
stress, 55, 272
  and Bernie's Ten-Point Plan for Health and Vitality, 39, 45
  emotional well-being and, 290–92, 294, 296, 298–99, 302
  fertility and, 130
  heart disease and, 238, 241–42
  hot flashes and, 77–78, 81, 87, 90
  NAS and, 209, 212–13
  osteoporosis and, 200
  and pregnancy in later life, 101
  and risk of early menopause, 29
  sexual enjoyment and, 178–80
sun, avoidance of, 268–69
support stockings, 279
surgery:
  in birth control, 114–18
  fertility and, 125–26, 140–41
  for gynecological cancers, 256–60
  hot flashes caused by, 87–88
  for hyperthyroidism, 230–31
  for male infertility, 149
  and risk of early menopause, 28
  see also specific surgical procedures
Synerol, 86
synthetic salmon calcitonin (SCT), 204
syphilis, 168

tamoxifen, 85, 98
teeth, protection of, 280–81
testosterone, 82, 150, 188

Index

thrombophlebitis, 60, 244–45, 278
thyroid and thyroid disorders, 4, 8, 23, 215–33, 290
  and aging, 21, 216
  and Bernie's Ten-Point Plan for Health and Vitality, 33–34
  diagnosis of, 224–27
  and hot flashes, 88
  how it works, 219–24
  and physical appearance, 263
  and PMS, 21
  risk of, 231–32
  and sex, 217, 220–24
  signs and symptoms of, 217–18
  treatment of, 227–31
thyroid scans, 227
thyroid stimulating hormone (TSH), 34, 47, 219–20, 223–25
thyroxine (T_4), 33, 88, 219, 225, 227–29
tight underwear, 147
Tofranil, 86–87
toxic shock syndrome (TSS), 107
transitional women, 3–24
  age-related experiences of, 17–21
  biological markers common to, 11–12
  counteracting common complaints associated with, 4
  Eskin's expertise on, 7–8
  key points about, 3–4
  prevalence of, 11
  psychological and psychosocial changes in, 22–24
  special needs of, 3
  who they are, 9–24
trichomoniasis, 166–67, 170
triiodothyronine (T_3), 219–20, 225
tubal ligations, 114–16

ultrasound, 45
  FCD and, 196
  fertility and, 142, 153
  fibroids and, 164
  male infertility and, 146

  for thyroid disorders, 226
  transvaginal, 260
urinary tract infections, 128
uterine cancer, 43
  menstrual changes and, 53–54, 61–62, 67, 75
  EST and, 67–68
  IUDs and, 113
  reducing risk of, 257
  treatment of, 256–57

vagina, 14
  atrophy of, 161, 173–74
  dryness of, 12, 16, 21, 31, 34–36, 74, 88, 109, 160–61, 173–74, 222
  keeping it in good shape, 161–63, 174
  menstrual changes and, 53, 74
  sexual enjoyment and, 160–66, 168–69, 171–73
vaginismus, 171–72
vaginosis, 166–67, 170
varicose veins, 278–79
vasectomies, 117–18
vision, aging and, 13–14
visualization, 302–3
vitality:
  Bernie's Ten-Point Plan for Health and, 30–47
  natural ways to maximize, 25–47
  and risk of early menopause, 26–30
vitamins, 20
  and Bernie's Ten-Point Plan for Health and Vitality, 40–42
  FCD and, 196
  gynecological cancers and, 251, 256
  heart and, 241
  for hot flashes, 90–91
  menstrual changes and, 56
  osteoporosis and, 201, 203
  physical appearance and, 266, 269, 273, 275

Index

waxing, 276
weight control, 5, 56
   and Bernie's Ten-Point Plan for Health and Vitality, 37–42
   birth control and, 109
   emotional well-being and, 284–85, 296–98
   fertility and, 130
   guidelines for, 37–38
   gynecological cancers and, 257
   heart and, 239, 241–43
   hot flashes and, 84
   loss of, 9–10
   and risk of early menopause, 27
   thyroid disorders and, 215–18, 224

varicose veins and, 279
wellness tests, 46–47
wrinkles, 22, 25, 45, 264, 286
   minimization of, 267–71

Xanax, 86–87

yeast infections, 165–66, 170
yoga, 304

zona drilling, 155
zygote intrafallopian transfer (ZIFT), 154–55

About the Author

BERNARD A. ESKIN, M.D., is an internationally renowned scientist in several areas of women's medicine. A pioneer in the field of reproductive senescence, he has helped to clarify the role of sex hormones in female aging. He writes and lectures widely on female sexuality. His book, *The Menopause: Comprehensive Management*, is in its third edition and is the leading clinical text on the subject. Dr. Eskin is a professor of Obstetrics and Gynecology at the Medical College of Pennsylvania and Hahnemann University. He is an editorial consultant for the *Journal of the American Medical Association*.

LYNNE S. DUMAS is the author of *Talking with Your Child About a Troubled World* and the coauthor of *Congratulations! You've Been Fired*. A journalist and social researcher, she has written for many national magazines including *Working Mother*, *Family Circle*, and *Woman's Day*.